PAIN

NEW PERSPECTIVES IN
THERAPY AND RESEARCH

PAIN

NEW PERSPECTIVES IN THERAPY AND RESEARCH

Edited by

Matisyohu Weisenberg
University of Connecticut Health Center
Farmington, Connecticut

and

Bernard Tursky
State University of New York
Stony Brook, New York

PLENUM PRESS · NEW YORK AND LONDON

Library of Congress Cataloging in Publication Data

Main entry under title:

Pain.

   Based on a sumposium—workshop at the annual meeting of the American
Association for the Advancement of Science, January 1975.
   Includes index.
   1. Pain—Congresses. 2. Analgesia—Congresses. I. Weisenberg, Matisyohu,
1936-   II. Tursky, Bernard.   III. American Association for the
Advancement of Science.
RC73.P34   616'.047   76-40023

ISBN-13:978-1-4684-2306-8   e-ISBN-13:978-1-4684-2304-4
DOI: 10.1007/978-1-4684-2304-4

Softcover reprint of the hardcover 1st edition 1976

Based on a symposium—workshop held at the annual meeting of the
AAAS, New York, New York, January 1975

© 1976 Plenum Press, New York
A Division of Plenum Publishing Corporation
227 West 17th Street, New York, N.Y. 10011

Preface

With the growing realization that pain and its control are vital areas for both theoretical and practical research as well as clinical treatment has come the desire for an assessment of the state-of-the-art. Pain research by itself is not new. Yet, approaches to the study and control of pain are new. This book is based upon a symposium-workshop on the study and control of pain that took place at the annual meeting of the American Association for the Advancement of Science, January, 1975. It was designed to deal with a number of theoretical and clinical issues. We attempted to assess previous years of research, how conceptions of pain phenomena have changed and what are some of the gaps in our knowledge. Presentations were also geared to show our increased methodological sophistication. Clinically, we have also changed our treatment conceptualization of pain control. We have not merely added a few "tricks" to deal with pain. Entirely new approaches are now available. Viewing pain as a public health problem we find many areas of needed research that should be directed toward the epidemiology of pain, the reduction of fear of obtaining health care, and unmet treatment needs.

Obviously, this book cannot provide full, comprehensive treatment of all the issues involved. It can, however, provide the reader with an understanding of the current, major thrusts, new research and treatment goals in pain control.

Recognition and gratitude must be expressed to the many individuals and organizations who were involved in arranging this symposium and its publication. The National Institute of Dental Research and the American Society of Clinical Hypnosis provided the financial support to make the symposium possible. Beyond their financial support our special thanks go to Dr. Aaron Ganz of NIDR and to Drs. Kay Thompson of the American Society of Clinical Hypnosis, for their valuable encouragement and advice. Dr. Sholom Pearlman of the Uni-

versity of Colorado School of Dentistry and Secretary of
section R of the American Association for the Advancement
of Science provided assistance and guidance throughout the
symposium.   The help of Mr. James Mears and the staff of
AAAS must also be acknowledged with many thanks.   A special
expression of gratitude goes to our secretary, Marilyn Glenn,
who helped with the numerous tasks that go into such a pro-
ject.

Matisyohu Weisenberg   Bernard Tursky
Farmington, Connecticut   Stony Brook, New York

Contents

INTRODUCTION

During the past few years we have witnessed a burgeoning interest in the field of pain and pain control from both practical-clinical and theoretical perspectives. Professional organizations such as the American Dental Association have published guidelines on teaching comprehensive programs of pain control (1972), specialized facilities have been developed for treating patients with chronic pain or for treating patients who have terminal conditions in which pain control is a significant problem. Organizations such as the International Association for the Study of Pain, its regional chapters, and the journal Pain have been established as forums for communicating to the many different constituencies interested in pain and pain control.

These developments point to the growing realization that pain control is a significant problem that has not been dealt with optimally either from a practical-clinical point of view or from a theoretical-experimental perspective. The delivery of health care on a daily basis most often involves either the alleviation of pain or the inflicting of pain as a concomitant of the treatment process. Reliance only upon pharmacological or surgical control has not always proven to be the most successful means of dealing with pain. As a consequence, there has been needless suffering. Some percentage of patients avoid care altogether while others, especially those with chronic pain, make the rounds from provider to provider in an endless search and preoccupation with pain.

Aside from drug research, experimental and theoretical focus has been mainly upon the sensation of pain. Only in recent years have the questions of distress and suffering come into the laboratory. Sensory physiologists and psychologists have described pain as a sensation along with temperature and other cutaneous sensations. (c.f., Geldard, 1972; Mountcastle, 1974). Emotional and motivational fac-

1

tors are usually mentioned as being very important in affecting the pain reaction. However, the major focus quickly
shifts back to such variables as the qualities of pain, the
nervous pathways involved in the sensory discrimination and
location of pain and the mapping of body sensitivity. Yet,
from a clinical perspective relieving pain may involve reducing the emotional-motivational components of pain while
the sensory aspects of pain are left unaltered (c.f., Casey,
1976).

Recent emphasis upon distress and suffering has been
helped by the increasing interaction of clinician and experi-
mentalist so that each can become familiar with the problems
of the other. This has included the acceptance of a multidisciplinary view of pain control with no single discipline
having all the answers and each discipline being able to
contribute its expertise to the unravelling of pain mys-
teries. This symposium was held in that spirit. It has
focused upon the latest approaches and issues in the clini-
cal-practical and in the theoretical-experimental domains.
Hopefully, each area will gain from the other.

Bonica (Chapter 1) and Shealy and Shealy (Chapter 2)
describe some of the current approaches as seen in the new
pain control centers that deal with chronic pain. Bonica
views the pain center as a place where all the available
knowledge regarding pain control can be made available in an
organized fashion to provide patient care, teaching and research. The University of Washington clinic brings together
13 different disciplines. Membership is based upon special
interest in chronic pain and the willingness to spend time
and effort utilizing unique skills in the diagnosis and
treatment of chronic pain problems.

While the Director is charged with providing overall
leadership, the Clinic Coordinator is given responsibility
for day-to-day patient flow. Each patient is assigned to a
physician who serves as Patient Manager. The Patient Manager is responsible for conducting the initial examination,
coordinating consultations and for providing the summary at
a patient case conference. Where a clear diagnosis exists
patients are referred for care. When the diagnosis is not
clear, the patient and spouse are asked to participate in
the multi-disciplinary case presentation to decide on a
course of action.

The pain clinic has become not just a place where patients are treated, but a focus for teaching medical students, residents and special fellows. It has also served as a stimulus for the conduct of pain research.

The LaCrosse program of Shealy and Shealy treats some 400 pain patients per year. The emphasis of the program is on behavioral and mechanical techniques as opposed to pharmacological, surgical or nerve block procedures. Shealy and Shealy advocate the use of autogenic therapeutic methods that include biofeedback, autogenic verbalization and physical exercise. It is felt that patients require from 6 to 12 hours of practice of these techniques each day for 2 to 4 weeks for about 25 percent of the pain population. The rest of the pain population may require 6 to 10 months of practice. The program is designed on an outpatient basis to teach patients pain control and not provide a cure. Much of the practice is done by the patient at home. Other clinic techniques used include acupuncture, external electrical stimulation, ice cubes and massage, and for some patients, facet rhizotomy.

Kutscher (Chapter 3) describes the unique problems of pain associated with the terminal patient. Newly formed treatment facilities such as Hospice are developing approaches for dealing with pain that allow the patient to maintain contact with reality and continue to respond to his/her environment. Death must not be viewed as a symbol of the physician's defeat. When cure is no longer possible, pain control may be one of the last realistic hopes. From the patient's point of view a terminal condition has often led to abandonment. Pain expression and complaint can be viewed by the patient as a reason for maintaining contact, while uncontrolled pain can increase the feeling of abandonment. Maintenance of personal dignity and freedom from pain without unnecessary drugging, therefore, reduces the fear of abandonment. Although pain control involves a multidisciplinary team, there is a feeling that there should be one individual who maintains patient contact at some greater level of intimacy. Terminal pain control thus includes drugs, surgery, hypnosis, acupuncture and most essential psychosocial approaches. The patient is assured of human contact. With time the variety of pain control approaches that are being tried undoubtedly will begin to make themselves felt in pain control in general, not just for the

terminally ill. All long-term pain-control techniques will
surely be affected.

One of the ancient procedures that has recently received a great deal of publicity is acupuncture. Three basic
theoretical approaches have been formulated. The traditional
Chinese approach describes acupuncture as working through a
series of body meridians to correct an imbalance of bodily
humors. Kroger (1973) has argued that acupuncture is nothing
more than hypnosis. He claims that he personally has carried out a great deal of surgery with hypnosis and can demonstrate similar phenomena. Spiegel, too, has called acupuncture needle hypnosis (personal communication). He
claims that his eye roll technique equally can determine if
a patient would benefit from hypnosis or acupuncture. Both
operate on the same principles.

Chaves and Barber (Chapter 4) discuss acupuncture in a
similar manner to their prior discussions of hypnosis in
surgery (c.f., Chaves and Barber, 1974). They feel that a
number of factors are overlooked in reports of the effectiveness of acupuncture as used in China. There is a selecti-
vity in choosing patients. Those that are chosen to have
surgery using acupuncture believe it will work. They are
also especially prepared in advance. As a consequence, the
selected patients have less anxiety. Narcotics, sedatives
or other drugs are used in combination with acupuncture.
The pain of surgery is less than most people assume. The
needles are also a form of distraction that provide the
suggestion of pain relief.

The results of a recent study by Goldberger and Tursky,
(in press) further complicate our understanding of the
effects of acupuncture. Experimental subjects received electrical acupuncture over correct loci with the suggestion that
the treatment would sensitize the area to the pain of electric shock. Control subjects received treatment at loci
that were inappropriate for acupuncture but with explicit
suggestion of analgesia. Comparison of reactive measures
showed that the experimental group, despite countersugges-
tions, showed increased threshold ratings for shock discomfort, pain and pain tolerance compared to the control
subjects. This effect persisted after acupuncture stimulation was discontinued. Magnitude estimation procedures,
however, showed no difference between groups.

Exactly what acupuncture is and how it works is not yet known. Clinically, however, even if it is nothing more than a variation of hypnosis, it can be extremely useful in pain control. For hypnosis, as Thompson (Chapter 5) points out, can be a significant means for dealing with pain problems. Thompson describes hypnosis as an altered state of consciousness in which the individual has an increased capacity to accept suggestion. Through hypnosis it is possible to remove the feeling of suffering and dread that can accompany such things as dental treatment. Although hypnosis is not a substitute for medical and surgical procedures, it can enhance the effectiveness of these procedures. The worst possible outcome with hypnosis is that nothing happens. At best, however, it can be a very powerful means of controlling pain.

One of the newer methods for teaching behavioral pain control is biofeedback training. Stroebel and Glueck (1973) have proposed that biofeedback is a form of placebo treatment. That is, the individual himself/herself in reality possesses the power for control. Biofeedback makes this ability explicit by permitting the person to actually experience control over bodily functions that may normally be relatively difficult to control. Stroebel and Glueck (Chapter 6) discuss biofeedback training for relief of tension and migraine headache. They propose that biofeedback can successfully prevent pain onset. It cannot eliminate pain after its onset. This generalization may not be valid, however, for other kinds of pain such as myofascial pain-dysfunction (personal patient treatment experience).

Conservative treatment strategies such as reassurance explanation, advice for self-management, psychological counseling, placebos, tranquilizers, etc. have been used by Greene and Laskin (Chapter 7) in their treatment of myofascial pain-dysfunction (MPD) patients. Use of surgery or extensive equilibration procedures was carefully avoided. MPD symptoms include muscular spasms and fatigue and have been viewed by Greene and Laskin as caused by emotional stress rather than by mechanical factors. An analysis of long-term treatment effectiveness as reported by patients after 6 months to 8 years showed that 51 percent had no recurrence of MPD symptoms since treatment. Another 41 percent had occasional minor episodes of pain but could

manage adequately. Only 6 percent reported that their pain
was not under control. Greene and Laskin feel that regardless of the treatment strategy tried for MPD, the most important factor was the doctor-patient relationship. Good
rapport and explanation of the problem seem vital. Undoubtedly, there are other pain syndromes for which a similar
statement can be made. The implication would be to spend
a little more time at interpersonal relationships and be a
little more hesitant in the use of surgical procedures.

How widespread in the population are the various problems of pain and pain control? Rayner (Chapter 8) deals
with this problem. The literature does seem to indicate
that pain and fear of pain do influence the willingness of
patients to seek health care. Pain can both motivate as
well as deter patients in seeking care. Exactly what percentage of the population is included is not clear. In
dentistry there are estimates of 9-15 percent of the population not seeking care because of fear of pain. For other
disease entities there are few statistics available. What
percentage of the population have chronic pain problems of
one kind or another is also not known at this time. These
public health issues certainly deserve a great deal more
attention than they currently receive.

The great emphasis upon doctor-patient relationships
and the use of behavioral techniques of pain control pre-
supposes that health care personnel are knowledgeable of
their value and can apply them in practice. Yet, Weisenberg
(Chapter 9) points out that examination of the few curricula
that exist for teaching pain control emphasize mainly pharmacological and surgical procedures. Nowhere are the behavioral and social aspects of pain fully developed. Weisenberg describes a multidisciplinary course on pain control
designed to teach a comprehensive view of the pain reaction.
The course reviews social, psychological, pharmacological
and physiological dimensions of the reaction to pain. Aside
from the didactic sessions, there are laboratory sessions
in which students can acquire knowledge and experience in
the use of behavioral techniques such as hypnosis, relaxation and biofeedback in pain control. Given the central
importance of behavioral techniques it would seem desirable
to expand such teaching efforts to allow students to feel
more comfortable in using alternative strategies in pain
control and thus rely less only upon medication and surgery.

The impetus for the recent emphasis on behavioral controls for pain has come largely through the gate-control
theory of pain perception (Melzack and Wall, 1965, 1970).
Whether the theory is "true" or not it has legitimized behavioral and psychological procedures by its view of pain
as a complex sensory and motivational phenomenum. Melzack
(Chapter 10) reviews many of the issues with which it has
tried to deal. These include the lack of a one-to-one re-
relationship between pain stimulus and pain response and
clinical phenomena as phantom limb pain and causalgia that
occurs with tissue healing and not tissue damage. Pain reactions also differ as a function of cultural grouping.

Neurophysiological evidence indicates a complex picture
that supports the concept of separate sensory and motivational nervous systems for pain perception. Recent studies
have also shown that stimulation of selected areas of the
brain stem can be effective in producing analgesia without
affecting sensory function.

The gate-control theory has recently come under a great
deal of criticism. Dyck, Lambert and O'Brien (Chapter 11)
present some of the evidence that is being used against it.
Gate-control theory has proposed that small fibers open the
gating mechanism and thereby increase pain stimulus transmission while large fibers close the gating mechanism and
thereby decrease pain stimulus transmission. In pathological conditions such as Fabry's disease where there is a
selective loss of large fibers patients have pain. In
Friedreich's Ataxia there is a selective loss of large
fibers and patients do not have pain.

Obviously, the gate-control theory will undergo modification. It was never intended to be complete by itself.
Currently it has both its proponents and its opponents who
seem to be viewing much of the same evidence as either supporting or opposing gate-control. If nothing else, gate-
control has certainly been a stimulus for increased pain
research and changes in clinical treatment strategies.

Laboratory research on pain control demands the placement of individuals in unpleasant conditions. Pain stimulation levels can often be high. It would be very helpful to
conduct research with animal populations. Dubner, Beitel
and Brown (Chapter 12) have developed an animal model that

utilizes intact organisms and is sensitive to motivational
changes that are independent of the sensory stimulus.

One of the most difficult and important tasks associated with pain control is reliable and valid measurement of
the many factors that enter into pain reactions. Tursky
(Chapter 13) has developed techniques that separate reactive
and sensory components using two different types of tasks.
The reactive measure asks subjects to respond to pain stimulation at four points: 1. sensation threshold, 2. discomfort, 3. pain and 4. tolerance. The sensory measurement
technique uses magnitude estimation in which a series of
pain stimuli are compared to a standard. Verbal measurement techniques have also been identified that allow for
the creation of scales that have been cross-modally validated.

Clark (Chapter 14) describes the use of sensory decision theory in pain measurement. This approach distinguishes between differences in perceived sensation and
differences in the criterion for labeling a stimulus as
painful.

Both the Tursky and Clark approaches have had and will
continue to have an impact on pain measurement. They allow
for a clearer evaluation of intervention strategies. That
is, does an individual perceive the pain stimulus as unchanged but is now unwilling to call it painful, or has a
particular intervention also changed the sensory discrimination of the pain stimulation as well.

These chapters have highlighted some of the major
developments in the study of pain and its control. We are
hopeful that such interchanges between researchers and
clinicians will inspire each to even greater effectiveness
in dealing with the important issues of pain control to the
benefit of all who suffer.

Matisyohu Weisenberg   Bernard Tursky

REFERENCES

American Dental Association, Council on Dental Education. Guidelines for the teaching of pain and anxiety control in dentistry. *Journal of Dental Education*, 1972, 36, 62-67.

Casey, K.L. Physiological mechanisms of pain perception. In M. Weisenberg (Ed.) *The control of pain*. New York: Psychological Dimensions, Inc. 1976.

Chaves, J.F. and Barber, T.X. Hypnotism and surgical pain. In T. X. Barber, N. P. Spanos and J. F. Chaves (eds.) *Hypnosis, imagination and human potentialities*. New York: Pergamon Press, 1974.

Geldard, F.A. *The human senses*. New York: John Wiley and Sons, 1972.

Goldberger, S.M. and Tursky, B. Modulation of shock elicited pain by acupuncture and suggestion. *Pain*, 1976, in press.

Kroger, W.S. Acupunctural analgesia: its explanation by conditioning theory, autogenic training and hypnosis. *American Journal of Psychiatry*, 1973, 130, 855-860.

Melzack, R. and Wall, P.D. Pain mechanisms: a new theory. *Science*, 1965, 150, 971-979.

Melzack, R. and Wall, P.D. Psychophysiology of pain. *International Anesthesiology Clinics*, 1970, 8, 3-34.

Mountcastle, V.B. Pain and temperature sensibilities. In V. B. Mountcastle, (Ed.) *Medical Physiology*. Saint Louis: C. V. Mosby, 1974.

Stroebel, C.F. and Glueck, B.C. Biofeedback treatment in medicine and psychiatry: an ultimate placebo? *Seminars in Psychiatry*, 1973, 5, 378-393.

ORGANIZATION AND FUNCTION OF A MULTIDISCIPLINARY PAIN CLINIC

John J. Bonica

University of Washington School of Medicine

Seattle, Washington

Although acute pain is useful because it compels patients to seek medical counsel and serves as a useful diagnostic aid to the physician, in its chronic pathologic form
it has no biologic value. Rather, chronic pain is a malefic
force which often imposes severe emotional, physical, and
economic stress on the patient, on his family, and on our
society. Although accurate statistics are not available,
data from a variety of sources suggest that chronic pain
states cost the American people between 50 and 75 billions
of dollars annually in hospital and health services and
loss of work productivity. Even more important is the cost
in terms of human suffering: millions of patients do not
get the relief they deserve. Many of these are exposed to
a high risk of iatrogenic complication from improper therapy,
including narcotic intoxication and multiple, often useless,
and at times mutilating operations; a significant number
give up medical care and consult quacks who not only deplete
the patient's financial resources but often do harm; some
patients with severe intractable pain become so desperate
as to commit suicide.

These deficiencies, which seriously detract from our
biomedical scientific achievements, are due to many causes
which have been detailed elsewhere.[1] Foremost among these
is the improper or inadequate application of knowledge
currently available and essential to proper management of
complex pain problems. These, in turn, are due to lack of
organized teaching of health professionals and the progressive trend toward specialization, which is conducive to

11

each specialist viewing pain in a very narrow, tubular fashion. In dealing with such complex pain problems, it is
often necessary for the patient's physician to enlist the
aid of one or more medical specialists and health professionals. One of the most efficient methods of managing patients with such problems is through the team approach and
through the multidisciplinary pain clinic, composed of
health professionals of different disciplines. Although I
proposed this concept over a quarter century ago and subsequently described it in many publications,[2] until recently
it was virtually ignored by the health professions. During
the past five years there has been a remarkable surge of
interest in this team approach and multidisciplinary pain
clinics have been organized in several medical centers
throughout the world. In this presentation I will briefly
summarize the evolution, organization, and function of one
such clinic at the University of Washington. A more detailed description is found elsewhere.[1,2,3]

EVOLUTION AND CURRENT STATUS

     Experience with military personnel during World War II
and, subsequently, with civilian patients led to the firm
conviction that the management of patients with complex pain
problems is best achieved through the well-coordinated and
concerted efforts of several health professionals who contribute their individualized knowledge and skills for the
common goal of making a correct diagnosis and planning the
most effective therapeutic strategy. In the immediate post-
war period, Alexander[4] proposed a similar concept and, for
a time, directed such a group. During the ensuing dozen
years I was successful in putting this concept into practice
in a community hospital and in 1961, in collaboration with
Dr. Lowell White, a neurosurgeon, founded the Pain Clinic
at the University of Washington. Subsequently, we invited
and gradually attracted psychiatrists, orthopaedists, psychologists, surgeons, and a variety of other specialists.
Qualifications for membership in the clinic included:
(a) special interest in chronic pain and the willingness to
spend sufficient time and effort; and (b) special knowledge
of pain syndromes and possession of unique skills to contribute to the diagnosis and therapy of chronic pain problems.

Currently the Pain Clinic group is composed of 20 individuals representing 13 different disciplines: anesthesiology, general practice, neurology, neurosurgery, nursing, oral surgery, orthopaedics, pharmacology, psychiatry, psychology, radiology, sociology, and surgery. The goals and missions of this group are: (a) to work as a well-coordinated team to provide optimal care to patients with chronic pain problems; (b) to carry on an effective teaching program for undergraduate, graduate, and postgraduate health professionals; and (c) to encourage independent and collaborative basic and clinical investigation. While these objectives can be achieved through individual efforts, our experience suggests that the team approach is more efficient and productive.

ORGANIZATION

A key to the success of such complex multidisciplinary efforts is in effective organization of the personnel and ample physical facilities, equipment, and financial resources. The organization of our own group is shown in Figure 1.

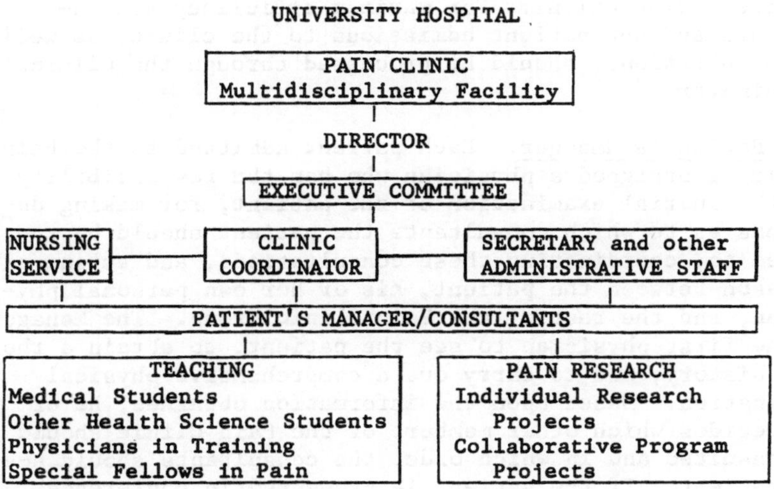

UNIVERSITY HOSPITAL

PAIN CLINIC
Multidisciplinary Facility

DIRECTOR

EXECUTIVE COMMITTEE

| NURSING SERVICE | CLINIC COORDINATOR | SECRETARY and other ADMINISTRATIVE STAFF |

PATIENT'S MANAGER/CONSULTANTS

TEACHING	PAIN RESEARCH
Medical Students	Individual Research Projects
Other Health Science Students	Collaborative Program Projects
Physicians in Training	
Special Fellows in Pain	

FIGURE 1. Organizational chart of the Pain Clinic

Personnel

Directors. The Director should have the capability of
providing vigorous medical, scientific, and administrative
leadership to the group. Since the team is composed of individuals who have appointments (and consequently allegi-
ance) to their parent departments, it is essential that the
Director possess those qualities necessary to bring a hetero-
genous group together and have it function as a single, efficient unit. He must possess a superior knowledge and
skills in a special area of pain and his performance in patient care, teaching, and research must be such as to accrue
him the respect of all his colleagues. We have an Assistant Director with similar qualifications who acts as a
backup for the Director and devotes most of his professional
time to the Pain Clinic.

Clinical Coordinator. The Clinical Coordinator acts
as the agent of the Directors and the entire group. To be
effective, this person must be able and willing to devote
most of his or her professional time to coordinate the functions and activities of the Pain Clinic. In addition to the
day-to-day patient care activities, this person must coordinate plans for the teaching programs and the scheduling
of case presentations. For maximum efficiency all in-
patients and out-patient admissions to the clinic, as well
as consultations, should be processed through the Clinical
Coordinator.

Patient's Manager. Each patient admitted to the Pain
Clinic is assigned a physician who has the responsibility
for the initial examination of the patient, for making decisions as to which consultants the patient should be referred to, coordinating these consultations, and acting as
a liason between the patient, his or her own personal physician, and the rest of the Pain Clinic Group. The Manager
is the first physician to see the patient, to obtain a thor-
ough history, and to carry out a comprehensive physical
examination. Based upon the information obtained, he or
she decides which other members of the Pain Clinic should
be consulted and in which order the consultants should see
the patient. If the patient is presented in conference,
the Manager (the house officer) presents a summary of the
patient's work-up to the group and after the conference he
relays the recommendations of the group to the patient and

to the referring physician. The Manager also has the responsibility of writing progress reports and follow-up of
the case.

Consultants. Consultants are individual medical specialists, usually members of the Pain Clinic Group, who devote a significant portion of their clinical time to the
care of patients with chronic pain. As previously mentioned,
in order to be members of the Pain Clinic Group they must
have special interest in and ample knowledge of pain syndromes and must possess specialized diagnostic and therapeutic skills in a particular field.

Health professionals other than physicians whom we consider essential to the success of this type of effort include dentists, oral surgeons, clinical psychologists,
pharmacologists, neurophysiologists, sociologists, and nurse
specialists with a particular interest in pain. These individuals serve in the same capacity as Consultants and
often provide valuable information which is not available
from other Consultants.

Other Personnel. Resident physicians who rotate
through the Pain Clinic, Special Fellows in Pain, and other
health professionals assigned to the Clinic as part of their
training constitute an important cadre of personnel which
helps with the work-up and day-to-day care of these patients.

The Pain Clinic Group should have ample secretarial and
administrative personnel. Because of her interface with the
public and her position in taking care of details of clinic
visits and admissions, the Secretary is among the most critical members of the group. Apart from acting as a routine
secretary to the members of the Clinic in their correspon-
dence, medical records, and referrals, the Secretary is
available during regular office hours to handle phone calls
and inquiries from physicians in the community.

Space and Equipment

To function optimally, the Pain Clinic Group requires
ample space and equipment of three varieties: (a) space in
the out-patient clinic, including a sufficient number of
large examining rooms fully equipped to permit a

comprehensive examination, several smaller rooms for return
visits, and a large room equipped to carry out special diagnostic procedures, including nerve blocks; (b) in-patient
beds, preferably within one ward or one area of the hospital,
staffed by specially trained nurses; and (c) specialized
space and equipment to meet the peculiar needs of a team
actively engaged in patient care and teaching. This includes a large theatre-type conference or lecture room for
the weekly conference, ample space and equipment for stor-
age and retrieval of patient records, and a variety of mechanisms for optimal communication among the members of the
Group and with the public.

FUNCTION

Patient Care

The Pain Clinic of the University of Washington accepts
only patients referred by physicians. Usually the patient
is referred to a specific member of the Pain Clinic Group,
but a significant number are referred nonspecifically to
the program. The function of the group is summarized in
Figure 2.

Procedures for Admission. Upon receipt of a request
to admit a patient the referring physician is asked to send
a summary of all the diagnostic and therapeutic procedures
done to date, including x-rays, operative reports, etc. He
or she is informed that the patient will be placed on a
waiting list pending receipt of the information and evaluation of the data by the Clinical Coordinator, who then decides whether or not the patient is a suitable candidate
for care by the group. The information not only helps
screening the patients, but also avoids excessive delay for
the out-of-town patients who otherwise will need to wait
while their records are being collected. Once the screening is completed and a decision is made to accept the patient, the referring physician and the patient are notified
of the appointment date. In many cases the patient is
asked to keep a two-week diary on a special form supplied
by the Pain Clinic, pertaining to drug medication and daily
activities, including "up-time" (the amount of time the patient is up and active) and "down-time" (the amount of time
the patient is in bed or inactive).

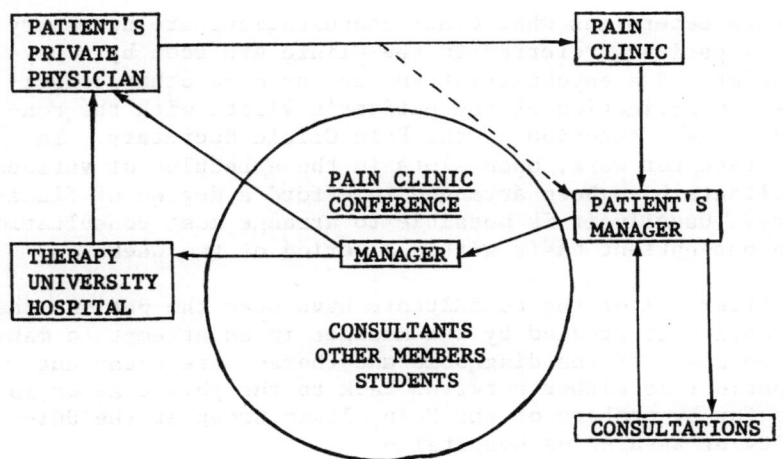

FIGURE 2.   Patient flow at the Pain Clinic

The Initial Visit. Those patients referred to specific
members of the Clinic are seen by them, who then become
their "managers." Patients who are not referred to a specific physician are assigned a Manager by the Assistant
Director. At the time of admission the patient is asked to
prepare a two-page description of the pain and family history on a special form and also complete the Minnesota
Multiphase Personality Inventory (MMPI) form. The information is then reviewed by the patient's Manager and subsequently the patient is seen and informed in detail about the
procedure of the Clinic work-up and how the Clinic functions.
A very detailed history of the pain and of the patient's
past medical history, family history, home and work environment, and other pertinent information is obtained. This is
followed by an examination of the painful region and general
physical examination, and usually a neurologic and ortho-
paedic examination. Usually the patient is then seen by a
nurse practitioner (Ph.D.), who carries out a sociologic
evaluation, and a social worker. Frequently, the initial
visit consumes 3-4 hours or longer.

The information is evaluated by the managing physician,

who then determines what other consultations are necessary.
Usually patients referred to the Clinic are seen by a psy-
chologist and a psychiatrist and one or more other consultants. Coordination of the patient's visits with the consultants is a function of the Pain Clinic Secretary. To
facilitate her work, open slots in the schedules of various
consultants have been arranged to afford a degree of flexi-
bility. Usually it is possible to arrange most consultations
on an out-patient basis within a period of two weeks.

After all of the consultants have seen the patient the
information is studied by the Manager in an attempt to make
a diagnosis. If the diagnosis and therapy are clear-cut,
the patient is either referred back to the physician or is
cared for by members of the Pain Clinic Group at the University of Washington Hospital.

The Conference. Patients in whom the diagnosis or therapy or both are uncertain are presented at the weekly conference of the Pain Clinic Group. Usually two patients are
considered during each conference, which lasts 1-1/2 hours.
The conference is chaired by the Director or Assistant Director. The patient's Manager or his House Officer presents
a summary of the history and physical findings and then calls
upon the consultants who have seen the patient to provide
additional information. Members of the Clinic who have not
seen the patient are given an opportunity to ask questions
and make comments.

The patient and spouse are then brought into the room
for further questions by members of the Clinic, including
those who have not seen the patient previously. The patient
and spouse are also given an opportunity to ask questions.
After this is completed, the patient and spouse leave the
conference room and there is further discussion among members of the Clinic. Often the discussion is vigorous and
continues until there is a consensus about diagnosis and
therapeutic strategy. After the conference, the patient's
Manager sees the patient and informs his or her of the decision made by the group. He advises the referring physician as soon as possible about the medical details of the
decision.

Experience has confirmed our deep conviction that this
face-to-face group discussion is more effective and

productive in making a correct diagnosis and formulating
the appropriate therapeutic strategy than communication by
letter or telephone or through fragmented independent efforts
inherent in traditional medical practice. In addition to
providing highly specialized consultant service to the referring physician and the patient, these conferences serve
as an excellent forum for exchange of ideas and information
and thus constitute a highly effective teaching mechanism.

Teaching and Research

The Pain Clinic carries out teaching programs for residents from various disciplines and for Special Fellows of
the Pain Service. Some of the medical students also rotate
as part of an elective clerkship. Residents usually rotate
for a period of one to two months while Special Pain Clinic
Fellows are accepted for periods ranging from three months
to a year or more. In addition to the clinical experience
on a preceptee-preceptor basis, they receive formal courses
and training by members of the Pain Clinic and are expected
to carry out some form of pain-related research.

During the early years the collaborative efforts of the
Pain Clinic Group were devoted exclusively to patient care
and teaching. Members of the group carried out independent
research in their own laboratories. However, with the participation of psychologists, pharmacologists, and other
basic scientists and clinical investigators there began
interaction, cross-fertilization, and communication which
has resulted in collaborative research. This has been one
of the most gratifying "spin-offs" of the group's activities.
For example, it was the early observation and participation
in the Pain Clinic Conference which prompted Dr. Wilbert
Fordyce to develop plans for a study of operant conditioning
principles to the management of patients with chronic pain.
Similarly, Dr. C. Richard Chapman's observation and experience in the Pain Clinic prompted him to radically revise
his approach to psychologic studies on pain. As a corollary,
the contribution of basic scientists has prompted a re-
vision of older concepts and the adoption of new ones in
regard to diagnosis or therapy or both. For example, Dr.
Lawrence Halpern was instrumental in prompting study of
drug intoxication as a major contributing factor to chronic
pain behavior.

REFERENCES

1. Bonica, J.J.: Organization and function of a pain clin-
        ic, in Bonica, J.J. (Ed.): International Symposium
        on Pain (Advances in Neurology, Vol. 4), New York,
        Raven Press, 1974, pp. 433-443.
2. Bonica, J.J.: The Management of Pain, Philadelphia,
        Lea & Febiger, 1953.
3. Bonica, J.J., and Black, R.G.: The management of a pain
        clinic, in Swerdlow M.: Relief of Intractable Pain.
        Amsterdam, Excerpta Medica, 1974, pp. 117-129.
4. Alexander, F.A.D.: The control of pain, in Hale, D.
        (ed.): Anesthesiology, Philadelphia, F.A. Davis
        Company, 1954.

BEHAVIORAL TECHNIQUES IN THE CONTROL OF PAIN: A CASE FOR HEALTH MAINTENANCE VS. DISEASE TREATMENT

C. Norman Shealy and Mary-Charlotte Shealy

Pain Rehabilitation Center

LaCrosse, Wisconsin

In a country which spends millions of dollars each year on drugs, medical care and hospitalization, isn't it ironic that so little attention is paid to PREVENTION? One cannot deny that disease treatment has made great strides in many areas over the years; in fact, the need for many disease treatments has been virtually wiped out by that very effective preventive tool, vaccination. Communicable disease control could make even more dramatic strides, however, were society in general and medical practitioners in particular HEALTH ORIENTED rather than disease-centered. Traditional medical care, including needless hospitalization, often results in little improvement in the patient's condition; in fact, exposure to an unfamiliar environment and other factors may trigger infections, drug reactions and other complications which worsen the patient's situation.

Most individuals consult a doctor only when they become symptomatic; 75 percent of the time the physician takes his diagnosis on the basis of history and physical examination. Even with the aid of the multitudinous diagnostic tests that he may use, some rather risky, the physician is diagnostically accurate at initial hospitalization only about 80 percent of the time. While a physician may attempt to eliminate the patient's disease problem, more often he is able only to treat the patient symptomatically.

In 60-85 percent of the symptoms presented, the underlying
problem is psychosomatic or psychophysiologic.

This dilemma in medical care is naturally vulnerable
to the reputed panacea, "druggism." Some years ago, tranquilizers descended upon physicians in endless array and
drug company advertisements promised miraculous results by
the bottleful of pills, the ampule or in oral liquid preparation, something for everyone every way! Tranquilizers,
starting first with THORAZINE^R, have become the most common
symptomatic therapy today. As mood modifiers, they have
had far-reaching effects among social relationships; one
can only speculate on the incredible modifications they may
have made on society as a whole. Drug companies spend 750
million dollars per year proselytizing physicians, providing
a major part of the post-graduate "education" of physicians.
The tranquilizer is a tantalizing temptation to the physician who feels he has exhausted unsuccessfully the alternatives for conventional medical treatment, and the patient
goes away, bottle in hand, feeling that the doctor has
"done something." Meanwhile in the past 25 years, pharma-
ceutical companies have become the most powerfully effective force in American medicine; their executives are the
highest paid group in the country; their profits are in the
oil industry league, a good share of the profits being
plowed back into the sales effort. Probably largely because
of this situation, psychophysiology's message is muffled
virtually unheard.

Disease-oriented care is generally charged for on a
fee-for-service basis; the tab is usually picked up by
third party carriers, led by Blue Cross-Blue Shield. Since
most insurance companies refuse to pay for outpatient
treatment, expensive hospital facilities have doubled in
the past twenty-five years as increasing numbers of people
seek insurance coverage, and subsequent medical care.

Another system of medical care, the Health Maintenance
Organizations (HMO), has also flourished in the past twenty-
five years. HMOs were started by the west coast-based
Kaiser company as an attempt to cut medical costs among
employees; the facilities have expanded to the general
public as the Kaiser-Permanente system. Although some routine examinations are done among participants in the plan,
HMOs are still primarily geared to treating dis-ease

(albeit earlier) rather than promoting health maintenance, i.e. illness prevention. For instance, little or no time is spent in introducing to patients the foundation of health maintenance, the principles of sound nutrition (except as disease-oriented diets for diabetics, for example); the Mormons and Seventh Day Adventists have done a much better job at promoting good health through the practice of wholesome nutritional habits and exercise than any medical system. Most doctors are abysmally ignorant of nutrition, thanks to medical schools which are primarily disease oriented. The proper promotion of health maintenance could be even more lucrative for insurance companies than disease treatment. Drug companies, tranquilizer-oriented physicians and other industries catering to a symptomatic society would lose in vast and gratifying ways. While such a turnabout in perspectives would require remarkable effort and cooperation among many media and individuals, the savings in lives, money, and general social disruption make the prospect of a health-oriented society very exciting and attractive.

Despite the limitations of today's HMOs in health maintenance, some rather interesting medical experience statistics give more than a hint of the possibilities inherent in a truly health oriented organization. In comparing HMOs with the Blue Cross system, they are separated as follows:

1. Blue Cross-Blue Shield (and other insurance plans) is a fee for service system.
2. HMOs are a prepayment plan for disease treatment.

The incidence of hospitalization is twice as great in the Blue Cross system as in the HMO plan. Furthermore, in 1966 there were 73 surgical procedures per 1000 population among Blue Cross-Blue Shield patients, as compared with merely 31 per 1000 patients in a comprehensive HMO plan. Tonsillectomy was 4 1/2 times as great in the BC-BS series; hysterectomies were twice as high, but more serious operations such as cholecystectomy were "only" 25 percent more common in the BC-BS patients. All this suggests "beyond any reasonable doubt," as the law likes to say, that surgery is related to the fee-for-service principle. It is, of course, also related to the incidence of surgeons. This is especially true in back surgery which correlates with an

area's census of orthopedists and neurosurgeons. Estimates
of excesses in back surgery range from 50 to 90 percent.

     No less an official than Dr. Peter Rogatz, Vice Presi-
dent of Blue Cross-Blue Shield of New York, emphasized in
a PRISM article, October 1974, that overutilization of hospital beds accounts for burgeoning health costs. Ironically,
Dr. Rogatz does not add that the in-patient treatment con-
tingencies of his company have been largely responsible for
the increases of which he complains!

     In one survey of an excellent general hospital, be-
tween 40 and 50 percent of patients were judged not to
require hospitalization. They were there primarily to
obtain insurance payment. This practice clearly is the
greatest single contributor to medical costs today. When
we consider the excesses of surgery widely reported, and
the overuse of drugs with their inherent complications (one
survey reported that 25 percent of patients were hospital-
ized because of complications of therapy, surgical and
medical), obviously the total health bill (and taxpayer
drain) could be strikingly reduced by a new direction in
health care, applicable to many problems.

     Dr. Lawrence L. Weed, originator of the problem-orient-
ed records system, commented in MEDICAL GROUP NEWS, July
1974, that medical knowledge is passed along like middle
age ballads. Dr. Weed, Professor of Medicine at the University of Vermont, believes that ours is a "lousy system" in
which over-diagnosis, over-treatment and over-medication
"are killing American Medicine." (Not to mention the
patient, though Dr. Weed did not say that.)

     There is great emphasis in medical rhetoric upon the
scientific advances of the American systems. Indeed, in
the management of ACUTE illnesses, advances are tremendous.
Treatment of bacterial infections, accidents and heart
attack victims are mostly scientific, remarkedly better
than 30 years ago and among the best in the world. The
medical world stumbles badly, however, when managing most
chronic diseases, especially psychosomatic problems; therapy
is erratic, often non-scientific and frequently ineffective
if not dangerous. One problem is that physicians either
don't have the time or don't take the time to develop a
rapport, a sense of trusted communication with the patient;

pitifully little attention is paid in medical schools to
the importance of psychological attunement as a vital component of successful patient care. For example, a busy
practicing gynecologist-obstetrician was questioned once
about his management of teen-age patients who came in for
sexual counseling. He replied, "I never bother talking
with them. I don't think they really want to talk. All
they need is The Pill, and they all get it." The Pill, a
drug of diverse and well known dangers becomes a substitute
for counseling and adult guidance among the community's
teenagers. Is it any wonder that the incidence of headache,
stroke and fertility problems, not to mention intractable
venereal disease, has soared among young people? Yet,
teen-agers who have the opportunity for honest counseling
in sexuality and alternatives to The Pill have often opted
for safer means of coping.

Tranquilizers are a cop-out too. While in acute situations tranquilizers can be of valid use, for long-term
purposes, they are not therapeutic. Tranquilizers snow the
mind and prevent the patient from coming to grips with his
problems. Some make a patient suicidal or seriously depressed while supposedly doing exactly the opposite. Over
the long term, they may have serious physiologic effects.
In any event, tranquilizers are the opposite extreme of
maintenance of good health; they don't even treat a disease
effectively.

To demonstrate the ramifications and possibilities of
a sound health maintenance program vs. a disease-oriented
system, the definition and discussion of chronic pain and
its management provides an ideal focus. Since pain is the
most common presenting symptom among patients (headache and
backache outweigh all other symptoms combined), it seems
appropriate to concentrate on this specialized symptom
complex.

Chronic pain is that which continues even though treatment of the original physical cause has been completed.
Ideally, pain should be a symptom, warning the patient that
tissue damage is possible. Although this is true in acute
pain, chronic pain is much more deceptive. Most chronic
pain is the result of already damaged nerve tissue and is
perpetuated by:

1. Scar, which restricts movement and which may

occasionally constrict nerves.

2. Sensory deprivation, in which the normal balance between pain and non-pain fibers is upset.

3. Faulty nerve regeneration, for example:

   a. A damaged skin nerve normally activated by pressure regrows to an end-point in a muscle. Every muscle contracture in that area is then interpreted as excess pressure or pain.

   b. Autonomic nerve fibers normally supply blood vessels and glands. When cut, they may regrow to attachments on bone, etc. and this sets up a perpetual barrage of misinformation, regional dysautonomia, etc.

4. The complex psychological disturbance associated with chronic illness.

In any of these situations, the invalid status invoked by chronic pain and repeated failure of therapy is markedly aggravated by the emotional disturbance of an altered life style. Frustration, anger, paranoia, and depression are easy to understand. Uncertainty and fear just as certainly contribute to hypochondriasis and hysteria. Furthermore, it is so likely that these personality traits will be distorted by chronic illness and suffering that patients remaining relatively stable become suspect! Most important, THE PATIENT REALLY DOES HURT! Writing him off as a hypochondriac or hysteric immediately interferes with his chances for developing a positive attitude or learning to cope with and hopefully allay his pain.

For most of this century, desperate chronic pain patients have been referred to neurosurgeons for consideration of surgery aimed at obliterating pain pathways. The excitement generated by the great work of Frazier in the early days of these procedures has never completely waned. Except for tic douloureux, some thoracic pain and unilateral cancer pain, however, the major destructive surgical procedures have been remarkably unsuccessful. In fact, despite the obvious failures including inability to relieve pain and unacceptable risks of neurological damage, two of the procedures, rhizotomy and cordotomy, led to the establishment of "pain clinics" at most medical schools and major medical centers.

Typically, the <u>traditional</u> pain clinic is "multidisciplinary." This implies that each patient is extensively evaluated by specialists in orthopedics, neurosurgery, anesthesia, neurology, physical medicine, psychiatry, social services, etc. In fact, each patient is screened by a gaulighter or triage manager who decides what specialists should actually see each patient. Usually the patient is pigeon-holed early in his evaluation, and therapy by one specialist is recommended. Only a small percentage of truly complicated patients are reviewed by the entire team. Treatment is usually surgical or traditional psychiatry. Many of the pain clinics specialize in nerve blocks, theoretically aimed at finding the exact nerve or group of nerves involved in transmitting pain. Inherently, such an approach supposes that pain can then be cut out or abolished by destruction of nerve pathways. Instead, the consequence of these procedures is frequently serious neurologic damage, leading to numbness, greater pain and other distressing symptoms such as impotence and incontinence. Even if the patient has been relieved of his pain, he may be unable to cope with the general inconveniences brought on by the procedure, and his general emotional status deteriorates markedly.

Most commonly, chronic pain, other than that caused by cancer, results from some disturbance in the back. For example, in the first 300 patients seen at The Pain Rehabilitation Center, S.C., LaCrosse (PRC), the ratio of back problems was 70 percent. Despite the large predominance of patients who represent back surgery failure, the only common etiology detectable to date is their membership in the species, Homo sapiens, which is peculiarly prone to back problems. Of 250 back surgery patients, only 8 had truly ruptured discs as revealed in the operative notes. In 42 patients the diagnosis was not obvious from description given; in 202 patients, surgery was undertaken solely because of the complaint of pain, but only a degenerated disc was found; surgery is not a cure for this problem. More disturbing, the average of these patients had had four unsuccessful surgeries. More is not necessarily better!

Most patients have had exhaustive attempts at drug therapy, psychotherapy, and at least serious consideration of destructive nerve surgery such as cordotomy, rhizotomy and cingulumotomy. Indeed, about 20 percent of these

patients have already had at least one of these procedures
by the time they present themselves to the PRC.

The total number of chronic pain patients in the United
States is unknown. Estimates range, however, from one
million to "an epidemic." If one considers the full range
of chronic pain problems involved in diseases such as arth-
ritis, moreover, the figures might tax the imagination.

The large collection of failures and complications of
traditional pain therapy has led in the past decade to new
approaches in the management of the chronic pain patient.
In 1966, for example, Dr. W. E. Fordyce brought operant
conditioning or behavioral modification to the pain field.
Patients with chronic pain problems are carefully selected,
25 percent of those referred being considered suitable can-
didates for the in-hospital program. Patients are evaluated for drug consumption, and ability to perform a half
dozen physical tolerance tests (sitting, walking, stationary
bike riding, etc.). During the approximate eight week program, patients are withdrawn from drugs by disguising them
in a liquid matrix, and gradually reducing the drug dosage.
Physical tasks are assigned on a progressive increase scale
beginning at a level below the patient's maximum tolerance.
As part of the psychological reinforcement program, patient's
complaints are ignored, while their performance successes
are praised. No adversive modification is used. Cost of
the eight week program was $5,000 as of 1971. Results have
been most encouraging. In the first five years of Fordyce's
program, 60 percent of 100 patients improved markedly. However, with a six month follow-up at least one third relapse
in the home environment. Despite the successes, one draw-
back in a program of this sort is that it is too small to
meet the vast supply of chronic pain patients seeking help.

In an effort to create an effective program which could
reach a greater number of patients, the first comprehensive
pain control program was begun in 1971 in LaCrosse, Wisconsin.[1] This approach, treating about 400 patients per year,
included behavioral modification, drug withdrawal, and a
variety of mechanical techniques directed at pain control;
more recently, PRC incorporated autogenics and biofeedback.
The mechanical pain relieving techniques are:

Acupuncture: quite useful in about 10 percent of patients. Some benefit is achieved in another 15 percent.

External electrical stimulation: about 25 percent of chronic pain patients find electrical stimulation helpful.

Ice: more useful than heat, ice rubdowns or Therapac[R] are effective in about 25 percent of patients.

Massage: both generalized and focal massage are a great help in creating relaxation, limbering and promoting a feeling of well-being.

Physical exercise: whether pain is relieved or not, most patients can increase physical activity to near normal, excluding heavy work. Scar can be stretched, and the patients can much improve their attitude and sense of well-being with increased exercise.

Facet "rhizotomy": a simple, safe electrical needle coagulation of nerves supplying spinal facets (the posterior vertebral joints often contributing to back and sciatic pain) is done under local anesthesia and is the most radical procedure still used. In 350 patients, marked pain relief (without any neurologic complications) has been achieved in 79 percent of backs not previously operated upon, 40 percent of those with previous surgeries and 25 percent of those with a fusion. Used in only 30 percent of the patients seen, the procedure has been the important, significant therapy in about 10 percent of the total 1100 patients treated.

Another vital component of the PRC program is autogenic therapy. The concept of autogenic therapy was introduced in 1932 by J. H. Schultz; later in his work, he collaborated with Wolfgang Luthe.[2] Together they have treated thousands of patients with their simple, auto-suggestive approach. While autogenic therapy has been reported to be useful in 80 percent of patients, particularly those with psychosomatic complaints, the techniques have not been widely used in this country.

Although almost 600 patients at the PRC have been exposed to autogenics, only 150 have had the intense 48 to 60 hours of instruction which has been used for the past year.

Chronic pain patients do not respond adequately to twenty
minutes of autogenics three times per day, as advocated by
Schultz.   The pervasiveness of the pain is responsible for
this problem.   Thus patients need 4 or more hours each day.

Another component of the PRC program is biofeedback
(BFB).   Dr. Elmer Green's reports of headache control
through biofeedback techniques (temperature for migraine,
EMG for tension) introduced a component of pain control
that ties in well with autogenics.   EMG, temperature, EEG,
and GSR are useful accessory reinforcements at the PRC,
particularly with headaches and in spinal paraplegia pain
syndrome.   Each of four paraplegic patients employing BFB
have controlled their long-standing (2 to 7 years) pain.
One 60 year old learned the technique in 48 hours, although
he continues to need practice.   A 20 year old required
about 6 months to reach 75 percent control of pain.

For optimal success, patients initially require about
6 to 12 hours a day of practice with BFB and autogenics to
gain control over pain.   About 25 percent of patients achieve
this control within 2 to 4 weeks; 80 percent of those patients who continue to practice the program at home achieve
control (not "cure") within 6 to 10 months.   In the past
six months, the PRC has used an intense outpatient program
to teach patients how to control pain rather than treat
symptoms.

Evaluation of pain is one of the most frustrating
tasks facing a dolorologist.   Drs. Picaza, Ray and Shealy
adopted a **Pain Profile** graded in each of 5 categories with
0 (normal) to 4 (maximum disability):

% of time pain present	0 – none
	1 – up to 25%
	2 – 26 to 50%
	3 – 52 to 75%
	4 – 76 to 100%
Severity of pain	0 – none
	1 – Mild
	2 – Discomforting
	3 – Distressing
	4 – Horrible or excruciating

Effect of pain on physical   0 - none
activity   1 - up to 25% incapacitated
                              2 - 26 to 50% incapacitated
                              3 - 51 to 75% incapacitated
                              4 - 76 to 100% incapacitated
Use of drugs   0 - none
                              1 - Aspirin and mild anal-
                                  gesics
                              2 - Tranquilizers and seda-
                                  tives in moderation
                              3 - Moderately addicting
                                  drugs - alcohol, code-
                                  ine, Darvon, Talwin,
                                  etc.
                              4 - Strongly addicting
                                  drugs - narcotics and
                                  large doses of those in
                                  No. 3
Effects of pain upon mood   0 - 4 (Panic; total incapac-
                                  ity)

The average chronic pain patients has a combined total score of 15 points (over 75 percent fall between 13 and 17) out of a possible 20 points maximum. Success of therapy is judged as fair to good if the pain profile is reduced by 30 to 50 percent, and excellent if the pain profile is reduced by 75 to 100 percent. This system of evaluation is the only one at present allowing comparisons among various therapeutic approaches.

Within a year after the PRC opened, other neurosurgeons began setting up similar programs in cities such as Portland, Boston, Omaha, and Indianapolis. Concrete plans are underway for a similar facility in Miami. Parts of the PRC system are in use in a number of cities. The use of intense autogenics should enhance all these programs.

Unfortunately, as pointed out earlier, over-hospital-ization is a problem in pain control programs because third party carriers such as BC-BS refuse to pay for outpatient care. Most chronic pain patients do not need hospitaliza-tion, the exception being severe drug addicts (about 10 per-cent of patients) who need withdrawal supervision. In fact,

most patients may progress faster if they are outside the
dependency environment of the hospital. The intense out-
patient program at the PRC suggests a possibility for a new
system of health maintenance.

Since 60 to 85 percent of all symptoms are psychosomatic or psychophysiologic, these symptoms should be treated
psychophysiologically. The only safe psychophysiological
system with adequate experience to date is autogenics.
Autogenics for purposes of this discussion consists of self-
motivated control of autonomic and physical symptoms.

Techniques include:

    Autogenic verbalization
    Biofeedback
    Physical exercise

Massage is an excellent reinforcing agent to other
techniques. Well-motivated patients who have a psychosomatic illness, anxiety or "nerves" would benefit from full
treatment by these techniques. Only in the 20 percent or
less who fail should other therapeutic approaches be considered. Obviously, this system requires a radical shift
in the focus of health care, for it implies that patients
would benefit from autogenic techniques for the control of
symptoms and, for the maintenance of health, as well as for
the treatment of illness. This is the ultimate in health-
maintenance and it requires patient self-responsibility.
Physicians would be less harrassed but freer for meaningful
patient communication, and complications of therapy would
drop dramatically. Some drug companies would go out of
business, but a solution to this latter problem is beyond
the scope of this paper!

A rational system to implement these techniques, in
the form of a series of autogenic training centers, Autogenics Pain Control and Health Systems is in the planning
stages under the sponsorship of a major insurance company.
APC-HS will teach autogenics techniques and progressive
physical exercise to the public. Even if it is only 80
percent effective in 70 percent of unhappy individuals (the
minimum average with psychophysiologic symptoms), it has
the potential for maintaining health and treating dis-ease
in a majority of Americans at a fraction of the cost of the
traditional systems.

REFERENCES

1. Shealy, C.N. The pain patient. <u>Am. Fam. Physician</u>,
        9:130-136, 1974.
2. Luthe, Wolfgang (Ed.), <u>Autogenic Therapy, Volumes I-VI</u>,
        Grune and Stratton, New York, 1969.

PAIN CONTROL AS A MULTIDISCIPLINARY PROBLEM

Austin H. Kutscher

Foundation of Thanatology, Columbia University
College of Physicians and Surgeons
New York, New York

Although today's section meeting is focused on the
control of pain, under a subsection designation of "dentistry," the topic of pain control is obviously one which tran-
scends the limitations of a specific discipline. Surely
head and neck pain from all causes, with our without mouth
pain, can be classified as a multidisciplinary problem. If
pain is to be considered from the viewpoints of new therapeutic approaches and frontiers for immediate research,
such avenues must be taken. The concept of pain control in
the terminal patient, therefore, demands an overview approach
and an overview conclusion, with the practitioner eschewing
any temptation to follow a middle of the road path that can
constrict clinical or research goals because of unproductive
tunnel vision.

There are fundamental similarities relating to pain
control of all terminal patients, regardless of anatomical
site of disease or the nature of the disease per se. On
the other hand, of course, counterbalancing differences
relative to the context of site and diseases and status of
the individual patient are also present. If one considers
regional pain only, one still must deal not only with such
overview factors as the primary disease state and its site,
alluded to in the above, but also, in addition, innumerable
other such factors including among many others, the patient's
physical and emotional status, the immediate cause and
severity of the pain, the moral and ethical issues associated with pain control procedures, the sociologic and
ethnic aspects of each particular situation, and a host of

interacting facets that involve the family and all manner
of caregivers vis a vis the patient himself.

A review of the titles of the papers presented at this
conference more than attests of this and the following:
that the NIDR (as well as nearly every branch of the NIH)
has a program on pain control; that new approaches in the
behavioral control of pain are being considered; that pain
control through the use of hypnosis is being subjected both
to a laboratory and a clinical review; that pain control
clinics are now in existence; and that, indeed, pain control
within the context of terminal care has found its way too
into this program. Other inferences within these titles
suggest the overview approach to terminal pain. These
would include the effect of health care organization on the
reduction of pain; the need to teach behavioral pain control
to health professionals; the basic science consideration of
the gate-control hypothesis; the structure of behavioral
animal models for the study of pain mechanism and control
as demonstrated by acupuncture; the fundamental issues of
clinical research and treatment for pain; and the community
or public health aspects of pain control. This particular
presentation will address itself to what is another broad
area--that of the psychosocial aspects of pain control in
the terminal patient and will interject certain philosophi-
cal comments and some of the practical questions raised by
these.

A primary result of effective pain control for the
terminally ill patient is the achievement of a major premise
of what is currently being called "death with dignity."
When the patient's pain is controlled properly, without
obtunding those other senses that keep him in touch with
reality, he can continue to respond to his environment, to
his caregivers, and to his family members with minimal de-
meanment and diminution of his normal role as an individual.
Contrariwise, the patient's pain, if ineffectually treated,
can adversely affect not only the patient but all of the
assemblage of professionals and involved people. The terminal patient has been described by others as being on a
trajectory toward death--which implies that this is an un-
remitting downward course. I would augment this: he is
also the hub of a circle that is transected by the reactions
of the many others on its periphery. If he is institution-
alized, hospital staff members surround him, reacting and

interacting with him; friends and family members visit to
maintain their interpersonal relations and emotional ties;
the medical staff, although finding it difficult to relin-
quish the struggle for care, tries to guide and manage his
care so that his dying becomes a meaningful part of his
living. Death should never be seen as a symbol of the physician's defeat, not by him nor by anyone else; the physician's dedicated effort on behalf of the patient who is dying can be a symbol of his having achieved the emotional
goal of "safe conduct," or in practical terms of having
successfully managed what has certainly been, in many instances, an almost unbearable clinical situation.

When cure is no longer a reasonable expectation, the
control of the terminal patient's pain is perhaps one of
his last two major realistic hopes. If this can be achieved
for him within his contracting fear-ridden world, it frequently enables the patient to rise above the totality of
his losses, suffering, and physical deterioration and even
to become a supportive presence for his family, his physician, and the other members of the caregiving team. Most
patients do not like to complain about pain as they are
fearful of upsetting those around them who find it difficult
to hear or see the effects of pain. Uncontrolled pain soon
leads to the abandonment of the patient by all who are of
significance in his life. Pain control permits the fulfillment of a second realistic hope of the terminal patient--
freedom from the actuality and/or the fear of being abandoned and lonely.

It should be stated parenthetically here that, although
it would be preferable if it were not so, the pain suffered
by the cancer patient is nearly always the target of clinical research models, to the exclusion of pain control in
those other diseases that account for more than 80% of
deaths. Each of these other causes would require, in its
model, differing factors that would take into account the
idiosyncracies of the illness and its incident pain, and so
forth, as alluded to above. Thus, in any brief presentation,
it is necessary to further compound the felony by considering pain control primarily in the terminal cancer patient
or those patients whose disease states bear resemblance to
the pain experience of cancer pain insofar as quality,
chronicity, intensity, etc. are concerned.

Within the area encompassed by the psychosocial aspects of pain control, we find ourselves most concerned with those people who are involved with or capable of influencing pain in general and the pain of the patient in particular.

Who are these people? A limited list would contain the patient himself, the family, the doctor, the nurse, the social worker, the volunteer, the housekeeper, the clergyman. To define this group in more specific terms, let us restate it as follows: the patient, the most immediate family member, close family members, distant relatives or relatives living at an emotional distance, the family practitioner, the primary care specialist be he surgeon or other specialist, the chief resident, others of the house staff, including the fast-disappearing intern, the terminal care specialist (chemotherapist, radiotherapist, etc.) the psychiatrist for the patient and/or family (also among the doctors), the RN, the nurse-specialist--extending to the terminal care nurse and the psychiatric nurse--, the licensed practical nurse, the nursing aide, the visiting nurse, members of the housekeeping staff (without forgetting the cleaning woman who I feel may have a truly valid conception of the patient's real condition, in many instances), the hospital social worker, the community based agency social worker, the homemaker, and others under the social service department; the candystriper, the gray lady, the escort service volunteer among this category of caregivers; and last, but by no means least, in this abbreviated listing, ministers who must fall into two categories--the hospital chaplain accustomed to facing and dealing with patient pain, and the parish minister, far less accustomed to dealing with physical pain but highly skilled at dealing with the pain of the human condition. This listing is concluded with the minister since he may be the nucleus of a team that must deal with the pain of those suffering anticipatory grief and, subsequently, bereavement while the doctor has primary control over the team dealing with pain in the hospital, especially in regard to the patient.

Are we stretching the point beyond relevancy when we include the painful sufferings of family and friends and caregivers in parallel with the physical suffering of the patient? I think not. And is the control of the former groups' emotional pain unrelated to the control of the patient's pain? Again, I think not. Each category of

caregiver is involved strategically with pain control,
though from a different perspective. Each has a different
armamentarium at his or her disposal, ranging from the most
potent narcotic-analgesics to tender loving care to silent
listening—all powerful weapons when brought into action at
the right time and in the right way. However, it should be
noted that within each category are numerous subgroups of
caregivers having unique and individualized approaches and
capabilities, as well as deficiencies that can detract from
the capacity to control the patient's pain. Also, in each
category of the above are the young and the old, the experienced and the inexperienced, the skilled and the unskilled,
the naturally talented and the innately inhibited, compris-
ing the whole spectrum of the human capacity and potential
to deal with pain.

The inability to bridge communication gaps can prevent
the proper use of pain control approaches that would be
simplified if these depended only on a one-to-one (doctor
to patient) relationship. But such is not usually the case.
The dying patient's lines of communication often carry his
messages of pain experience and his fears of pain to a nurse
and thence to a doctor; or to a family member to a nurse to
a doctor; or to a nurse to a family member to a clergyman
to a doctor—only then with a response back to the patient
and too often with inadequate action being taken to ease the
pain and the fear of it. The communications gap possibilities are exponential, tragically so; for as the line stretch-
es, the intimacy required to achieve pain control in all of
its dimensions is interrupted. Although a team approach to
care delivery for the terminal patient presents an excellent model, there must be ultimately individual patient-to-
caregiver contact at some level of intimacy. All too often
we do not know for sure who can give the patient the most
relief, or what combination of caregiver or caring talents
will prove to be the most ameliorative.

That terminal pain control is thus not exclusively determined by the analgesic action of a drug is in accord with
other cardinal factors: 1) the non-analgesic narcotic effect (or the improved patient affect) that is a major attri-
bute of narcotic analgesics in terminal pain control; 2) the
less often employed surgical, hypnotic, acupuncture, and
other techniques; and 3) the psychosocial approaches as
absolutely essential complements and supplements to all of

these. Such a conclusion is supported by, among other facts,
the widespread usage of imipramine and chlorpromazine, among
other agents of a mood altering nature employed in various
geographic locals, under widely diverse circumstances, by
practitioners holding widely divergent views regarding the
ideal to be sought as total pain control.

Now let us consider the following three provocative
problem areas, if we might: 1) the drug, heroin; 2) addiction; and 3) abandonment of the patient. The approach to
these will be facilitated if it can be accepted that at St.
Christopher's Hospice in London a philosophy of psychosocial
and physical care is being practiced that represents ideal-
ized terminal care. In one variation or another (the Hospice
being built in New Haven, for an almost replicated example,
or, conceptually, as a facility within other existing institutions such as is now being organized within St. Luke's
Hospital in New York), the St. Christopher "system" is being
introduced into this country. St. Christopher's serves as
a model for nearly every desirable aspect of terminal care:
where pain control is achieved--through the carefully controlled use of a drug, heroin, in this case; where abandonment of the patient is avoided; and where addiction is not
allowed to interfere unduly with the philosophic objects of
pain control for the patient, but where the psychopharmacologic know-how of the staff minimizes the theoretical and
practical concerns of addiction. This know-how is not beyond the reach of our practitioners.

A relationship with the patient begins as he enters the
hospice and is greeted by staff members; a contract is made
stating that he or she will be kept free of pain, or as
close to this as is humanly possible. The patient is thus
reassured that the dreaded and feared physical and mental
burdens of pain will be removed from his life. Though dying,
he will be allowed to live as a human, not as a drugged veg-
etable. From all the evidence--supported by data emanating
from the Hospice and by the reports of many neutral observ-
vers who have visited there from this country--this aspect
of the contract is effectively fulfilled. When daily ad-
justment of pain control agents is made with great care and
deliberation for each patient individually, when an around-
the-clock nurse-to-patient ratio, not often approached in
this country, is the rule, when numerous psychosocial modalities are contributed by others on the staff and by the

total family who all care for the patient, when the support
of religion is accorded the patient where this is of comfort, when emotional factors that can lower the patient's
pain threshold are routinely avoided--when these are the
elementary articles in the contract, not only is pain controlled but so too is the fear of and the actuality of
abandonment.

Whether or not the use of heroin in the British "cock-
tail" is an absolute condition to such effective control of
pain and abandonment is probably beside the point of whether
or not a pain-free and abandonment-free death with dignity
are feasible. (If concerns about addiction are brought into
the perspectives surrounding dying, then some other agent
other than heroin can be sought.) Currently, the British
are considering the relative advantages of heroin as compared with morphine; in this country we are working with
Levo-dromoran as opposed to morphine, in an attempt not only
to discern differences between these two agents but also to
see if Levo-dromoran possesses the prized mood altering
activity, so effectively implemented by heroin, within the
context of an adequate analgesic therapeutic index. If not
heroin or Levo-dromoran, then perhaps we must turn to agents
of similar potency for clinical trial, drugs which society
has not branded inacceptable on the sole basis of their (as
yet unproven) addictive liabilities.

Psychopharmacologic test models at the clinical pharma-
cologic and clinical research levels are available, are being used, and are constantly being adapted to evaluate with
greater precision the relief of the patient's physical and
emotional pain and the tempering of the effects of stress-
ful experiences on those who care and give care. Although
some in this country may flinch at the clinical dosage or
addictive liability of such dosages of narcotic analgesics
as may be needed to control a terminal patient's physical
pain and his emotional stress, the British model clearly
reveals that such totality of relief for patient, family,
doctor, nurse, friend, and all others who care is possible
within the context of avoidance of the induction of behavior incompatible with the terminal status of the patient
or the frame of mind or reference that most individuals and
society would deem to be inappropriate. Terminal patients
living in a state of dignity, such as those depicted above,
are realities. They are not having highs; they are not

looking for highs; they are looking simply for pain relief.
When pain is relieved, the patient's mood changes and he
becomes a sociable human being. Abandonment of the patient
is no longer to be feared, for, painfree, he will be eager
to maintain his contact with his environment and those significant others in this life can be expected to respond
when they have assurance that each visit to the bedside will
not be a painful experience for them.

Innumberable problems complicate the attempt to control
terminal pain; these will be dealt with as hypothetical
premises are tested. For example, at our medical center
the relative desirablility of staying ahead of pain with
drug therapy (another St. Christopher's approach) rather
than overcoming it upon each instance of its recurrence is
being explored. The model suggests the former approach to
be more appropriate from many viewpoints although it is not
completely within the bounds of traditional pain therapy.
It should not be difficult to confirm such an hypothesis.
And so on.

What in the end seems reasonably evident and a source
of positive speculation is the fact that if we would permit
our intellectual efforts and our technical expertise to be
teamed with our hearts and our spirits, two realistic hopes
may be achieved for the terminal patient: his pain will be
controlled and, concomitantly, he will not be abandoned by
those who are his caregivers and those who care enough to
be part of his every living moment. When pain control is
absent, the patient will most likely be treated as a dying
patient. However, when pain control is a reality, it will
be possible for everyone involved to treat the patient as
a living person--even though he is passing through the dying
process.

ACUPUNCTURE ANALGESIA: A SIX-FACTOR THEORY*

John F. Chaves and Theodore Xenophon Barber

Medfield Foundation and Medfield State Hospital

Medfield, Massachusetts

During recent years, physicians from the United States, Canada, and England have visited China and have observed the successful use of acupuncture to relieve surgical pain (Brown, 1972; Capperauld, 1972; Capperauld, Cooper and Saltoun, 1972; Dimond, 1971; Hamilton, Brown, Hollington and Rutherford, 1972; Jain, 1972a, 1972b; Shute, 1972; Tkach, 1972). These eyewitness accounts have produced widespread interest in acupuncture analgesia as indicated by many discussions in the popular press and also by a series of papers in medical journals (Chisholm, 1972; Liu, 1972; Mann, 1972; Matsumoto, 1972; Taub, 1972; Toyama and Nishizawa, 1972).

From Psychoenergetic Systems, 1:11-21, Copyright 1974, Gordon and Breach Science Publishers Ltd.   Reprinted by permission.

*This paper was presented at the Second Western Hemisphere Conference on Acupuncture, Kirlian Photography and the Human Aura, 1973, and is being published in a book based on that conference.   It is republished here with permission of the authors and publisher.

Work on this paper was supported by a research grant (MH-19152) from the National Institute of Mental Health, U.S. Public Health Service.   Early versions of this paper were presented by J. F. Chaves at the annual meeting of the Massachusetts Psychological Association, Boston, 12 May 1972, and at the Society for Clinical and Experimental Hypnosis, Boston, October, 1972.

At least part of the interest seems to be due to the implication that Western medicine cannot explain the efficacy of acupuncture in attenuating pain during surgery. The dramatic successes claimed for acupuncture seem to imply that Western science has failed to delineate important factors that pertain to the nature of pain and its control. We do not accept these implications. On the contrary, we believe that six factors which are already known but usually overlooked by Western medicine can help explain the success of acupuncture in relieving surgical pain. Three of these factors are:

a) the patients who are accepted for surgery with acupuncture strongly believe in its efficacy and are not fearful or anxious;

b) with few exceptions, narcotic analgesics, local anesthetics, and sedatives are also used, singly or in combination, during surgery with acupuncture; and

c) the pain normally associated with many surgical procedures is less than is generally assumed. Three additional relevant factors are that (d) the patients are typically exposed to special preparation and indoctrination for several days prior to surgery, (e) the acupuncture needles distract the patients from the pain of surgery, and (f) suggestions for pain relief are present in the acupuncture situation.

After we have briefly described the technique of acupuncture, we shall discuss each of these six relevant factors. Also, towards the end of the paper, we shall briefly discuss two popular theories of acupuncture - the traditional Chinese meridian theory and the more recent gate control theory.

TECHNIQUE OF ACUPUNCTURE

Although the use of acupuncture to treat specific illnesses such as arthritic disorders and gastrointestinal diseases goes back at least 5,000 years (Veith, 1972), its use to relieve the pain of surgery is very recent. In fact, the Chinese started using acupuncture to produce analgesia in surgery in 1959 and its use has accelerated since 1968 (Capperauld, 1972; Hendin, 1972).

During the 14 years that acupuncture has been used for surgical analgesia, the thin needles have been typically inserted at points that are remote from the location where analgesia is desired. For instance, when a gastrectomy is performed, four acupuncture needles are placed in the pinna of each ear. The needles are usually inserted only a few mm. and rarely inserted more than two centimeters beneath the epidermis. Moreover, they are commonly placed in innocuous locations such as in the limbs or the pinnae, remote from major organs, blood vessels, or nerve trunks. When acupuncture is used for surgery, the needles are not simply inserted; instead, they are either twirled and vibrated by the acupuncturist, or electricity is applied to them. Typically, continuous electrical stimulation is applied to the acupuncture needles from a 6- or 9-volt battery at a frequency of 120 to 300 cycles per minute, beginning about half an hour before and continuing throughout the operation (Dimond, 1971; Jain, 1972a). However, it is important to note that electrical stimulation does not appear to be essential to the success of acupuncture analgesia since many surgical procedures are performed using only manual stimulation of the needles.

It is generally assumed that if the acupuncture needles are inserted in the appropriate locations and are either twirled manually or electricity is applied to them, sufficient reduction in pain is produced so that the patient can tolerate major surgical procedures. Since the reduction in pain has been attributed to the effects of the needles, little attention has been focused on six other factors, to which we now turn, that may account for the apparent analgesia that is found in the acupuncture situation.

1. Strong Beliefs and Lack of Anxiety

The widespread assumption that acupuncture is routinely employed with surgical patients in China is false. The chief delegate of a group of Chinese physicians who visited the United States in the Fall of 1972, expressed concern

lest the Americans misunderstand (acupuncture analgesia as an established, standard technique in China (Anon. 1972).

Observations by Dimond (1971) indicate that,

> The decision to use acupuncture anesthesia depended
> on the full enthusiasm and acceptance by the patient.

Patients who are anxious, tense, or frightened are given
general anesthesia. Surgeons typically select patients for
acupuncture according to the following criteria:

> They decide whether the type of operation would be
> suitable, whether the patient would be too hysteri-
> cal, whether the patient believes firmly in Mao's
> teaching, or would Mao's teaching carry him through
> (Warren, 1972).

Since general anesthesia is available for surgery in China,
the motivation to forego general anesthesia and to undergo
surgery with acupuncture is probably due to the

> ...immense pressure to comply and participate in
> the current Mao Thought program which is a funda-
> mental requirement for life in China (Dimond, 1971).

Before surgery with acupuncture is commenced, the patient
and attending physicians recite quotations from Chairman
Mao's book and Mao's picture faces the patient in every
operating room (Jain, 1972a). Also, at the end of the
operation, the patients routinely thank Chairman Mao for
the surgery (Dimond, 1971).

Two additional points should be noted here. First, in
some localities in China, the insertion of acupuncture
needles is practiced by laymen in about the same way as
individuals in Western countries take aspirin tablets
(Capperauld, 1972). Capperauld (1972) has pointed out that
in some parts of China

> young children practice inserting needles into one
> another's arms, legs, and face to become proficient
> both as user and as a recipient.

Secondly, it should be emphasized that the Chinese
learn early in life to expect little or no discomfort dur-

ing surgery, even when the surgery is performed without
drugs and without acupuncture. For instance, Brown (1972)
states:

> While visiting a children's hospital we saw a queue
> of smiling five-year-olds standing outside a room
> where tonsillectomies were being carried out in
> rapid succession. The leading child was given a
> quick anesthetic spray of the throat by a nurse, a
> few minutes before walking into the theatre un-
> accompanied. Each youngster in turn climbed on the
> table, lay back smiling at the surgeon, opened his
> mouth wide, and had his tonsils dissected out in
> the extraordinary time of less than a minute. The
> only instruments used were dissecting scissors and
> forceps. The child left the table and walked into
> the recovery room, spitting blood into a gauze
> swab. A bucket of water at the surgeon's feet
> containing 34 tonsils of all sizes was proof of the
> morning's work. This tonsillectomy technique is
> significant inasmuch as it indicates that, without
> recourse to acupuncture, the Chinese patient is
> conditioned from early childhood to accept surgical
> interference with his body with the full knowledge
> that it is going to be successful and he will experi-
> ence little or no discomfort.

Kroger (1972) has appropriately summarized these points
by noting that

> Specific factors responsible for acupuncture
> anesthesia are: the antecedent variables such as
> the generalized stoicism of the Chinese, the ideo-
> logical zeal, the evangelical fervor, the prior
> beliefs shared by acupuncturists and patients (and)
> Mao Tse-tung's New Thought Directives....

Mann (1973) has recently provided further support for
the notion that the patient's belief in the effectiveness
of acupuncture is crucial to its success. Working in England, he attempted to use acupuncture to produce analgesia
to pinpricks in 100 volunteer subjects. Acupuncture failed
to produce satisfactory analgesia to the pinpricks, which

were severe enough to draw blood, in at least 90 percent of
these subjects. Mann attributed the tremendous discrepancy
between his success rate and the success rate reported from
China as due to the following: in contrast to the Chinese,
he did not attempt to lead his subjects to believe that acupuncture would be highly effective.

2. Use of Narcotic Analgesics, Local Anesthetics, and
    Sedatives

     Although popular accounts imply that narcotic analge-
sics, local anesthetics, and sedatives are not used when
patients undergo surgery with acupuncture, eye-witness
accounts from Western physicians do not support this notion.
Man and Chen (1972) state that, during surgery with acupuncture, the Chinese routinely administer 50 to 60 mg. of
meperidine hydrochloride (Demerol) in an intravenous drip.
Of the six cases described by Dimond (1971), three received
meperidine hydrochloride (50-60 mg.) intravenously during
their operations (a gastrectomy, a subtotal thyroidectomy,
and a removal of a thyroid adenoma). A fourth patient, who
underwent thoracic surgery, was given 10 mg. of morphine
subcutaneously. A fifth patient received a sedative dose
(0.2 gm.) of phenobarbital sodium together with subcutaneous
scopolamine (0.3 mg.) prior to surgery and intraperitoneal
local anesthesia (procaine hydrochloride) during the surgery (oophorectomy). A sixth patient recived phenobarbital
sodium the night before surgery; however, she did not receive pain-relieving drugs during the surgery (removal of
brain tumor) and, although she was described as "conscious,
but very weak," she tolerated the operation without signs
of pain. The latter case is indeed remarkable. However,
it should be noted that brain tissue is generally insensitive to the surgeon's scalpel (Lewis, 1942) and, in other
eye-witness reports of operations for cerebral tumor carried out with acupuncture, it is emphasized that the surgeons infiltrated the scalp with 50 milliliters of 0.125
percent procaine before the incision was made (Brown, 1972;
Capperauld, 1972).

     In his eye-witness report of surgery with acupuncture,
Capperauld (1972) noted that, typically, barbiturate medication was given preoperatively and meperidine hydrochloride
and promethazine hydrochloride were given intravenously
during the operation. After also noting the use of local
anesthetics, Capperauld (1972) asked,

The real question to be answered, therefore, is
which therapy, the acupuncture needle or the concomitant Western medication, is the adjunct?

Recent reports of surgery with acupuncture performed
here in the United States also note the use of narcotic
analgesics together with sedatives. For instance, Liu
(1972) reported a tonsillectomy carried out with acupuncture
on a nurse-anesthetist. The patient was given preoperative
medication (two ml. of Innovar) which included a narcotic
analgesic (fentanyl citrate) and a phenothiazine-like psycho-
sedative (droperidol). As Price and Dripps (1970) have
pointed out, this neuroleptic-narcotic mixture produces
"general quiescence and a state of psychic indifference to
environmental stimuli" and is useful in carrying out minor
surgical procedures. It is interesting to contrast this
tonsillectomy, performed in the United States with an analgesic, sedation, and acupuncture on a medically sophisticated patient, with the routine tons llectomies, without
analgesics, sedation, or acupuncture performed on Chinese
children.

It should be noted that, in some cases, the drugs that
are given during acupuncture fail to control pain, that is,
the patient complains of intolerable pain and general anesthesia is administered. Dimond (1971) estimated that this
kind of failure occurred in China in at least ten percent
of the selected patients. During a three-week visit to
China, Dr. Marcel Gemperle (1972) failed to find a single
case where acupuncture produced complete insensitivity and,
in one case, the patient screamed and moved about on the
operating table during surgery. As we noted earlier, Mann
(1973) found a failure rate of at least 90 percent in England
when no attempt was made to convince subjects of the effectiveness of acupuncture in reducing the pain of pinpricks.

3. Overestimation of Surgical Pain

Since, in Western medicine, anesthetic or analgesic
agents are now practically always used during major surgery,
there is little information regarding the baseline levels
of pain experienced by surgical patients who have not received pain-relieving drugs. However, even during the pre-
anesthetic era (prior to the 1840's), some patients

undergoing major surgery without drugs "bravely made no
signs of suffering at all" (Trent, 1946). For instance, in
one such operation (a mastectomy) carried out in the early
1800's, the patient tolerated the surgery

> ...without a word, and after being bandaged up,
> got up, made a curtsy, thanked the surgeon and
> walked out of the room (Freemont-Smith, 1950).

Although patients of this type probably represented only a
small minority of those undergoing surgery during the pre-
anesthetic era, they indicate the major importance of determining base levels of pain when evaluating procedures such
as acupuncture.

The available evidence indicates that surgical procedures produce anxiety and fear but they usually give rise
to less pain than is commonly believed. In summarizing the
relevant evidence, Lewis (1942) emphasized that, although
the skin is very sensitive, the muscles, bone, and most of
the internal organs are relatively insensitive. More precisely, the skin is sensitive to a knife cut, but the underlying tissues and internal organs are generally insensitive
to incision (although they are generally sensitive to other
forms of stimulation such as traction or distention). For
example, Lewis (1942) noted that the subcutaneous tissue
gives rise to little pain when it is cut and slight pain is
elicited when muscles are incised. Most of the internal
organs also produce little or no pain when they are cut;
these include the liver, spleen, kidneys, stomach, jejunum,
ileum, colon, lungs, surface of the heart, esophageal wall,
and uterus. Traction upon the hollow viscera, however, is
painful. Also, the surgeon's incision produces pain when
it cuts the skin and other external tissues (such as the
conjunctiva, the mucous membranes of the mouth and naso-
pharynx, the upper surface of the larynx, and the stratified
mucous membranes of the genitalia) and also when it cuts a
small number of deeper tissues (such as the deep fascia,
the periosteum, the tendons, and the rectum) (Lewis, 1942).
In brief, although "pain receptors" may be widely scattered
throughout the body, and although many tissues and organs
give rise to pain when they are stretched or pulled or
when pressure is applied, most tissues and organs of the
body (with the notable exception of the skin and other external tissues) give rise to little or no pain when they

are cut by the surgeon's scalpel.

In the early 1900's, Lennander (1901, 1902, 1904,
1906a, 1906b) published a series of case reports indicating
that major abdominal operations can be accomplished painlessly using only local anethetics, such as cocaine, to
dull the pain of the initial incision through the skin.
Mitchell (1907) also reported an extensive series of major
operations performed with local anesthetics that were used
to produce insensitivity of the skin. These included:
limb amputations, thyroidectomies, mastectomies, suprapubic
cystostomies, laparotomies, excision of glands in the neck
and groin, herniorrhaphies, cholecystostomies, and appen-
dectomies.

Mitchell (1907) confirmed Lennander's observation regarding the surprising insensitivity of internal organs.
For example, he noted the following:

> The skin being thoroughly anesthetized and the
> incision made, there is little sensation in the
> subcutaneous tissue and muscles as long as blood
> vessels, large nerve trunks and connective tissue
> bundles are avoided....The same insensibility to
> pain in bone has been noted in several cases of
> amputation, in removal of osteophytes and wiring
> of fractures. In every instance after thorough
> cocainization of the periostium, the actual mani-
> pulations of the bone itself have been unaccom-
> panied by pain. The patients have stated that
> they could feel and hear the sawing, but it was
> as if a board were being sawn while resting upon
> some part of the body.

The data presented by Lewis (1942), Lennander (e.g.,
1901), and Mitchell (1907) suggest that the pain associated
with major surgical procedures may not always be as great
as is usually supposed. It is certainly clear that the
amount of pain is not related in any simple way to the
extent of surgical intervention. Obviously, it is necessary
to have a base-line measure of pain in order to evaluate
the effectiveness of any procedure, including acupuncture,
that is said to produce analgesia. The evidence available
at present indicates that, if a patient is relaxed and not
anxious and if he can tolerate the initial incision through

the skin, many major surgical procedures can be accomplished
without much additional pain. The administration of small
or moderate doses of narcotic analgesics and sedatives, as
is usually done with acupuncture, makes the patient's task
that much easier.

Chinese surgeons who employ acupuncture, conduct their
operations very slowly and carefully (Brown, 1972; Capperauld, 1972). Rib-spreaders employed during thoracotomies
are opened slowly. Also, surgeons avoid putting traction
on such tissues as the pleura and peritoneum which are
known to be sensitive to traction (Brown, 1972). When these
tissues are stretched, acupuncture patients grimace, sweat,
and show other signs of experiencing extreme pain (Capperauld, 1972), just as would be expected on the basis of the
data summarized by Lewis (1942). Acupuncture is difficult
to use in abdominal surgery because it is hard to avoid
putting traction on these tissues and because acupuncture
does not produce adequate relaxation of the abdominal muscles (Jain, 1972a; Shute, 1972).

In brief, at least some of the success of acupuncture
in surgery can be accounted for by three considerations:
the patients strongly believe in the efficacy of acupuncture
and they are not fearful or anxious; narcotic analgesics,
local anesthetics, and sedatives are commonly used, singly
or in combination, along with the acupuncture; and most
tissues and organs of the body are insensitive when they
are cut. However, for a more complete explanation of the
success of acupuncture, three additional factors need to
be taken into account: the patients are typically exposed
to special preparation and indoctrination for several days
prior to surgery; the acupuncture needles distract the
patients from the surgery; and suggestions for pain attenuation are present in the acupuncture situation. Let us now
look at the latter three factors in turn.

4. Special Preparation and Indoctrination Prior to Surgery

Patients who are selected for surgery with acupuncture
receive rather special treatment preoperatively. The patient typically comes to the hospital two days before the
surgery and the surgeons explain to him exactly what they
are going to do, they show him just how they will operate,

and they explain to him what the acupuncturist will do and
what effects the needles will have (e.g., Jain, 1972b).
Also, the patient is asked to talk to other patients who
have had the same kind of surgery and he is given a set of
acupuncture needles so that he can try them on himself. As
Capperauld (1972) has pointed out,

> Acupuncture anesthesia tended to work better in non-
> emergency situations in which the patients had a few
> days indoctrination prior to operation. Emergency
> operations were done usually under conventional
> spinal techniques.

It thus appears that preoperative familiarization with the
medical setting and with the surgical procedures may play
an important role in further reducing any anxiety regarding
the forthcoming operation and in reducing the need for
large doses of pain-relieving drugs (Finer, 1970).

Although this kind of special preoperative preparation
and indoctrination for surgery is not employed in the United
States, there is evidence to indicate that "preoperative
education," even if very limited, can have a beneficial
effect on surgical patients. For instance, Egbert, Battit,
Welch, and Bartlett (1964), found that a five or ten minute
preoperative visit by an anesthesiologist had a greater
calming effect on surgical patients than two mg. (per kilo-
gram of body weight) of pentobarbital sodium. Moreover,
patients who were informed about the kind of post-surgical
pain they might experience required smaller doses of narcotics for post-surgical pain than uninformed controls. An
unexpected bonus was that the informed patients were dis-
charged from the hospital sooner than the controls.

In brief, it appears that the preoperative period of
special preparation and indoctrination for acupuncture
provides an opportunity to reduce further the patient's
anxiety, to strengthen his "belief and trust in acupuncture"
(Wall, 1972) and to reduce his need for large doses of
pain-relieving drugs.

5. Distraction Produced by Acupuncture Needles

The insertion and subsequent stimulation of the

acupuncture needles is accompanied by various sensations.
At times, the electric current that is applied to the needles is strong enough to produce rather strong muscular
contraction. Also, the needles are manipulated by hand or
stimulated electrically for 20 to 30 minutes prior to surgery and the patient often feels "sore" at the sites of
needle placement (Chen, 1972; Man and Chen, 1972). McGarey
(1972) noted that,

> A deep but minimal aching sensation is often felt
> when the needle is properly placed.

Some patients report that the acupuncture needles produce
severe pain. Mann (1973) found that, in order to reduce
the pain of pinpricks it was necessary, with most subjects,
to increase the pain produced by the acupuncture needles
"...to more or less torture levels." In describing his own
sensations while undergoing acupuncture for the relief of
post-surgical abdominal pain, James Reston (1972:8) noted
that the needles

> ...sent ripples of pain racing through my limbs
> and, at least, had the effect of diverting my
> attention from the distress in my stomach.

In brief, the acupuncture needles produce various sensations and they can serve as distraction. The evidence
available at present indicates that distraction is an effective method of reducing pain. Notermans (1966) found substantial (40 to 50 percent) increases in the threshold for
pain when subjects were distracted by performing an irrele-
vant task (inflating a manometer cuff). Kanfer and Good-
foot (1966) showed that pain could be reduced by three
types of distractors (observing interesting slides, self-
pacing with a clock, and verbalizing the sensations aloud).
Similarly, it has been demonstrated in several reports
(Barber, 1969a; Barber and Cooper, 1972; Barber and Hahn,
1962) that experimentally-induced pain could be reduced by
various kinds of distractions (listening to an interesting
tape-recorded story, adding numbers aloud, and purposively
thinking of pleasant events).

The distraction produced by counter-irritation is also
an effective way of reducing pain. Gammon and Starr (1941)
demonstrated that experimentally-induced pain could be

reduced by several kinds of counter-irritations including heat, cold, vibration, electric stimulation, and static electricity. Gammon and Starr (1941) also found that counter-irritation was effective in alleviating clinical pain. In one group of 60 clinical patients, 90 percent obtained some degree of relief from pain, although the most effective type of counter-irritation varied in different patients.

The studies cited above demonstrate that a wide variety of distractions are effective in attenuating pain. Clearly, the acupuncture needles themselves can serve as effective distractors. In addition, some acupuncture patients receive special deep breathing exercises which they later are requested to carry out during surgery (Brown, 1972; Warren, 1972). By focusing their attention on their breathing during the surgery, the patients may be provided with an additional useful distraction.

6. Suggestions for Pain Relief

It is clear that patients who are selected to undergo surgery with acupuncture believe that the technique is effective in attenuating pain. During the preoperative indoctrination and also during the surgery itself, the patients' pre-existing beliefs are strengthened by direct and indirect suggestions that acupuncture will mitigate pain. Even when acupuncture is used to treat specific diseases, Rhee (1972) noted that

...the acupuncturists whom I have watched work, load their therapy with suggestion.

The effectiveness of indirect suggestions in the clinical setting has a long history and has often been observed serendipitously. For instance, Tuckey (1889) wrote:

There are few cases of this kind more remarkable than one related by Mr. Woodhouse Braine, the well-known chloroformist. Having to administer ether to an hysterical girl who was about to be operated on for the removal of two sebaceous tumours from the scalp, he found that the ether bottle was empty, and that the inhaling bag was free from even the odor of any anesthetic. While

a fresh supply was being obtained, he thought to
familiarize the patient with the process by putting
the inhaling bag over her mouth and nose, and tell-
ing her to breathe quietly and deeply. After a few
inspirations she cried, "Oh, I feel it; I am going
off," and a moment after, her eyes turned up and
she became unconscious. As she was found to be
perfectly insensible, and the ether had not yet
come, Mr. Braine proposed that the surgeon should
proceed with the operation. One tumor was removed
without in the least disturbing her, and then, in
order to test her condition, a bystander said that
she was coming to. Upon this, she began to show
signs of waking, so the bag was once more applied,
with the remark, "She'll soon be off again," when
she immediately lost sensation and the operation
was successfully and painlessly completed.

Working under primitive conditions in a prisoner-of-
war hospital near Singapore, Sampimon and Woodruff (1946)
found, to their surprise, that "the mere suggestion of
anesthesia" was sufficient to perform minor surgery on the
soldiers without apparent pain. In a more recent report
from Bulgaria, Lozanov (1967) demonstrated that suggestions
of anesthesia are at times sufficient to carry out major
surgery with little pain. Similar findings have emerged in
studies of placebos. Hardy, Wolff, and Goodell (1952)
showed that pain thresholds could be elevated 90 percent
over control levels when an inactive drug was administered
with the suggestion that it was a strong analgesic. Moreover, placebos have been found to be effective in alleviating post-surgical pain and also chronic pain in many patients (Barber, 1959; Beecher, 1955; Dodson and Bennett,
1954; Houde and Wallenstein, 1953; Laszlo and Spencer,
1953).

Suggestions of anesthesia are also effective in attenuating experimentally-induced pain. Barber and Hahn (1962)
and Evans and Paul (1970) showed that suggestions of insensitivity attenuated cold-pressor pain. Similarly,
Barber (1969a) and Spanos, Barber and Lang (in press)
showed that suggestions of anesthesia reduced the pain
produced by a heavy weight applied to a finger. Using
the same pain stimulus on the finger, Chaves and Barber
(1973) found that the mere expectation of pain attenuation
led to a reduction in pain, although larger reductions

were obtained when subjects were asked to vividly imagine
that their finger was numb and insensitive or to imagine
pleasant experiences they had had.

Taken together, then, clinical and experimental observations indicate that both direct and indirect suggestions
of anesthesia are effective in attenuating pain (Barber,
1963, 1969b, 1970, 1972). It also appears likely that suggestions play a role in attenuating pain in the acupuncture
situation.

In summary, we have delineated six factors that help
to explain the efficacy of acupuncture in attenuating surgical pain. Surprisingly, none of these factors are taken
into consideration in the two most prominent theories of
acupuncture analgesia, the traditional Chinese meridian
theory and the more recent gate control theory. Let us
briefly examine these theories.

TWO PROMINENT THEORIES OF ACUPUNCTURE ANALGESIA

Chinese Meridian Theory

The traditional Chinese theory of acupuncture, which
has been described by Mann (1972) and Drake (1972), assumes
that there are 12 meridians (Ching lo) or channels running
vertically down the body. These meridians are thought to
carry a life energy (Ch'i, Ki, or Qi). The flow of this
energy is thought to maintain a balance between two forces,
the Yin and the Yang. Yin is viewed as the weak, female,
negative force, while Yang is the strong, male, positive
force. Yin meridians are associated with such organs as
the liver, kidneys, and spleen, while Yang meridians are
associated with such organs as the stomach, gall bladder,
and intestines. Disease is thought to reflect the imbalance of Yin and Yang forces. The insertion of acupuncture
needles in appropriate locations is thought to correct the
imbalance and thus cure the disease. Consequently, to produce analgesia for surgery, it is necessary to insert acupuncture needles into meridians which control the appropriate organs. Since the meridians are thought to run through
the whole body, the points of insertion may be quite remote
from the points where analgesia is desired.

Although this ancient theory of acupuncture still appears to have many advocates in China, it is not accepted by all Chinese surgeons. Man and Chen (1972) note that some Chinese surgeons "totally disregarded the recognized spots on the meridians" and used almost any spot to produce surgical analgesia. It thus appears that the traditional theory of acupuncture points may be misleading.

Mann (1972) who has written several books about acupuncture and who, at one time, accepted the traditional theory, now argues,

...I don't believe meridians exist. A lot of acupuncture is based on meridians, and you will see from my theory, I think the meridians of acupuncture are not very much more real than the meridians of geography. And likewise with the acupuncture points.

Mann (1972) goes on to note that

The Chinese have so many interconnections in their acupuncture theory that one can explain everything just as politicians do.

Wall (1972) is more succinct in his discussion of meridians, stating that

There is not one scrap of anatomical or physiological evidence for the existence of such a system.

Gate Control Theory

Several writers (Man and Chen, 1972; Shealy, 1972; Wall, 1972; Warren, 1972) have commented on the relevance of Melzack and Wall's (1965) Gate Control Theory of pain in understanding acupuncture analgesia. This has been, perhaps, the first attempt to apply a theory of pain that has any degree of acceptance among Western scientists. Briefly, the theory asserts that pain depends, in part, on the relative amounts of activity in large $\underline{A}$-beta fibers, activated by non-painful stimuli, and small $\underline{c}$-fibers, activated by pain-producing stimuli. Increasing the activity of the $\underline{A}$-beta fibers is thought to close a spinal "gate" in the substantia

gelatinosa, preventing the further transmission of information from the c-fibers. As applied to acupuncture, it is
assumed that acupuncture needles selectively stimulate the
A-beta fibers and that the high level of activity in the
A-beta fibers closes the "gate" and thus inhibits pain.

At first glance, the gate control theory may appear to
be more helpful than the six factors we have discussed in
accounting for anecdotal reports in the popular press which
suggest that acupuncture may be useful in performing surgery with rabbits, horses, and other mammals. Of course,
these statements in newspapers and magazines cannot be
evaluated until such time as non-anecdotal studies are presented which, at least, utilize minimal controls. Since
there is much evidence demonstrating that many mammals, including rabbits and horses, can tolerate extremely painful
stimuli when they are appropriately restrained (Ratner,
1967), controlled studies may find that acupuncture is not
especially helpful in operating on mammals.

There are major difficulties in using the gate control
theory to account for acupuncture analgesia. First of all,
the "gate" is a hypothetical entity that has not been established anatomically. Even if such a "gate" were shown
to exist, the gate control theory, as originally formulated,
could only account for analgesia in the vicinity of the
nerves stimulated by the acupuncture needles (Shealy, 1972;
Wall, 1972). However, as we noted earlier, acupuncture
needles are typically inserted at points which are remote
from the area where analgesia is desired. A related difficulty is that many of the locations commonly employed in
acupuncture, such as the head or pinnae, would be ineffective in closing the spinal "gate." Thus, it is necessary
to postulate the existence of a second "gate," presumably
located at some higher level of the nervous system, in
order to account for the efficacy of needles inserted at
these locations (Man and Chen, 1972). While it is difficult
to rule out this possibility, the postulation of new "gates"
on an ad hoc basis to account for anomalous findings is not
satisfactory.

As originally formulated, the gate control theory
appears inadequate to explain how acupuncture attenuates
the pain of surgery. Recently, Wall (1972), who is one of
the original co-authors of the gate control theory, stated

that

> My present guess is that...it will emerge that
> acupuncture does not generate the specifically
> pain-inhibiting barrages for which I was looking.

However, Melzack (1973a, 1973b), the other co-author of the
gate control theory, has recently argued that the theory is
relevant to acupuncture. While the gate control theory may
appear to be useful in explaining the successes of acupuncture, it is very difficult to see how this theory can
account for its failures. Why is it necessary for acupuncture patients to believe in its effectiveness? If acupuncture needles can close the "gate," why is it necessary to
administer narcotic analgesics, sedatives, and local anesthetics to acupuncture patients? Why is the "gate" capable
of reducing the pain of surgery in China, but incapable of
reducing the pain of pinpricks in England (Mann, 1973)?
Unfortunately, gate control theory fails to provide answers
to these important questions. It appears to us that speculations regarding the physiological basis for acupuncture
analgesia may be premature.

CONCLUDING COMMENTS

In this paper we have tried to take into consideration
the available data pertaining to surgery with acupuncture
analgesia. As more data become available additional factors
will surely be identified that will also help to explain
this phenomenon. It remains to be deomonstrated, however,
that acupuncture needles exert any specific analgesic effects beyond those indicated in the present paper. Certainly, future attempts to account for the success of acupuncture in attenuating surgical pain should take into
account the factors that we have delineated.

It appears to us that the success of acupuncture analgesia underscores the importance of psychological factors
in the control of pain. However, more research is needed
to determine the relative importance of the six factors
described in this paper and to identify additional factors
that could help to explain the phenomenon. Certainly, providing the basis for a more comprehensive explanation of
acupuncture analgesia will be an exciting area for future
research.

REFERENCES

Anon. China s doctors on tour. Medical World News, 1972, 13, 34-48.

Barber, T.X. Effects of hypnotic induction, suggestions of anesthesia, and distraction on subjective and physiological responses to pain. A paper presented at the annual meeting of the Eastern Psychological Association, Philadelphia, 1969a.

Barber, T.X. Hypnosis: A Scientific Approach. New York: Van Nostrand Reinhold, 1969b.

Barber, T.X. LSD, Marihuana, Yoga, and Hypnosis. Chicago: Aldine, 1970.

Barber, T.X. Suggested ("hypnotic") behavior: The trance paradigm versus an alternative paradigm. In Hypnosis: Research Developments and Perspectives (Fromm E., and Shor, R.E. (eds.). Chicago: Aldine-Atherton, 1972, pp. 115-182.

Barber, T.X. The effects of "hypnosis" on pain: A critical review of experimental and clinical findings. Psychosomatic Medicine, 1963, 25, 303-333.

Barber, T.X. Toward a theory of pain: Relief of chronic pain by prefrontal leucotomy, opiates, placebos, and hypnosis. Psychological Bulletin, 1959, 56, 430-460.

Barber, T.X. and Cooper, B.J. Effects on pain of experimentally-induced and spontaneous distraction. Psychological Reports, 1972, 31, 647-651.

Barber, T.X. and Hahn, K.W., Jr. Physiological and subjective responses to pain-producing stimulation under hypnotically-suggested and waking-imagined "analgesia." Journal of Abnormal and Social Psychology, 1962, 65, 411-418.

Beecher, H.K. The powerful placebo. Journal of the American Medical Association, 1955, 159, 1602-1606.

Brown, P.E. Use of acupuncture in major surgery. Lancet, 1972, 1, 1328-1330.

Capperauld, I. Acupuncture anesthesia and medicine in China today. Surgery, Gynecology and Obstetrics, 1972, 135, 440-445.

Capperauld, I., Cooper, E., and Saltoun, D. Acupuncture anesthesia in China. Lancet, 1972, 2, 1136-1137.

Chaves, J.F. and Barber, T.X. Cognitive strategies, experimenter modeling, and expectation in the attenuation of pain. Medfield Foundation Reports, 1973, No. 129.

Chen, J.Y.P. Acupuncture. In Medicine and Public Health
in the People's Republic of China (Quinn, J.R., ed.).
Washington, D.C.: U.S. Department of Health, Education
and Welfare, and National Institutes of Health, 1972,
pp. 65-90.

Chisholm, N.A. Acupuncture analgesia. Lancet, 1972, 2,
540.

Dimond, E.G. Acupuncture anesthesia: Western medicine and
Chinese traditional medicine. Journal of the American
Medical Association, 1971, 218, 1558-1563.

Dodson, H.C., Jr. and Bennett, H.A. Relief of postoperative
pain. American Surgeon, 1954, 20, 405-409.

Drake, D. Yin, Yang, and acupuncture. In Acupuncture:
What Can It Do For You? New York: Newspaper Enterprise
Assn., 1972, pp. 28-31.

Egbert, L.D., Battit, G.E., Turndorf, H., and Beecher, H.K.
The value of the preoperative visit by an anesthetist.
Journal of the American Medical Association, 1963, 185,
553-555.

Egbert, L.D., Battit, G.E., Welch, C.E., and Bartlett, M.K.
Reduction of postoperative pain by encouragement and
instruction of patients. New England Journal of Medicine, 1964, 270, 825-827.

Evans, M.B. and Paul, G.L. Effects of hypnotically suggested analgesia on physiological and subjective responses to cold stress. Journal of Consulting and
Clinical Psychology, 1970, 35, 362-371.

Finer, B. Physiological studies of the relationship between the doctor and the patient in pain. Acta Uni-
versitas Upsala, 1970, 1, 1-24.

Freedman, L.R. The relevance of acupuncture. Yale Journal
of Biology and Medicine, 1972, 45, 70-72.

Freemont-Smith, F. Discussion of Beecher's paper on perception of pain. In Problems of Consciousness, First
Conference. New York: Josiah Macy, Jr., Foundation,
1950.

Gammon, G.D. and Starr, I. Studies on the relief of pain
by counter-irritation. Journal of Clinical Investigation, 1941, 20, 13-20.

Gemperle, M. Cited in Science Digest, 1972, 73, 6.

Hamilton, S., Brown, P., Hollington, M., and Rutherford,
K. Anesthesia by acupuncture. British Medical Journal,
1972, 3, 352.

Hardy, J.D., Wolff, H.G., and Goodell, H. Pain Sensations
and Reactions. Baltimore: Williams and Wilkins, 1932.

Hendin, D. Is acupuncture today's medical miracle? In
    Acupuncture: What Can It Do For You? New York: News-
    paper Enterprise Assn., 1972, pp.4-7.
Houde, R.W. and Wallenstein, S.L. A method for evaluating
    analgesics in patients with chronic pain. Drug Addic-
    tion and Narcotics Bulletin, 1953, Appendix F:660-682.
Jain, K.K. Glimpses of Chinese medicine, 1971 (Changes
    after the cultural revolution). Canadian Medical As-
    sociation Journal, 1972a, 106, 46-50.
Jain, K.K. Glimpses of neurosurgery in the People's
    Republic of China. Internal Surgery, 1972b, 57, 155-
    157.
Kanfer, F.H. and Goldfoot, D.A. Self-control and toler-
    ance of noxious stimulation. Psychological Reports,
    1968, 18, 79-85.
Kroger, W.S. Hypnotism and acupuncture. Journal of the
    American Medical Association, 1972, 220, 1012-1013.
Kroger, W.S. More on acupuncture and hypnosis. Society
    for Clinical and Experimental Hypnosis Newsletter, 1972,
    13, (4), 2-3.
Laszlo, D. and Spencer, H. Medical problems in the manage-
    ment of cancer. Medical Clinics of North America, 1953,
    37, 869-880.
Lennander, K.G. Beobachtungen über die Sensilität in der
    Bauchhöhle. Mitteilungen aus den Grenzgebieten der
    Medizin und Chirurgie, 1902, 10, 38-104.
Lennander, K.G. Ueber die Sensibilität der Bauchhöle und
    über lokale und allgemeine Änasthesie bei Bruch- und
    Bauchoperationen. Centralblatt Für Chirurgie, 1901, 8,
    209-223.
Lennander, K.G. Ueber Hofrat Nothnagels zweite Hypothese
    der Darmkolikschmerzen. Mitteilungen aus den Grenzge-
    bieten der Medizin und Chirurgie, 1906a, 16, 19-23.
Lennander, K.G. Ueber lokale Änasthesie und über Sensi-
    bilität in Organ und Gewebe, weitere Beobachtungen.
    Mitteilungen aus den Grenzgebieten der Medizin und
    Chirurgie, 1906b, 15, 465-494.
Lennander, K.G. Weitere Beobachtungen über Sensibilität
    in Organ und Gewebe und über lokale Anasthesie. Deutsche
    Zeitschrift für Chirurgie, 1904, 73, 297-350.
Lewis, T. Pain. New York: Macmillan, 1942.
Liu, W. Acupuncture anesthesia: A case report. Journal
    of the American Medical Association, 1972, 221, 87-88.

Lozanov, G. Anesthetization through suggestion in a state
  of wakefulness. In Proceedings of the 7th European
  Conference on Psychosomatic Research. Rome: Privately
  printed, 1967, pp. 399-402.
McGarey, W.A. The philosophy and clinical aspects of acupuncture as viewed from the framework of Western medicine. In Transcript of the Acupuncture Symposium. Los
  Altos, Cal.: Academy of Parapsychology and Medicine,
  1972, pp. 12-22.
Man, P.L. and Chen, C.H. Acupuncture "anesthesia"--a new
  theory and clinical study. Current Therapeutic Research,
  1972, 14, 390-394.
Mann, F. The probable neurophysiological mechanism of acu-
  puncture. In Transcript of the Acupuncture Symposium.
  Los, Altos, Cal.: Academy of Parapsychology and Medi-
  cine, 1972, pp. 23-31.
Mann, F. Acupuncture anesthesia. A paper presented at the
  Symposium on Acupuncture, New York University School of
  Medicine, 1973.
Mann, F. Acupuncture: The Ancient Chinese Art of Healing.
  New York: Vintage Books, 1962.
Matsumoto, T. Acupuncture and U.S. medicine. Journal of
  the American Medical Association, 1972, 220, 1010.
Melzack, R. The Puzzle of Pain. New York: Basic Books,
  1973a.
Melzack, R. Why acupuncture works. Psychology Today,
  1973b, 7, 28, 30, 32, 34, 37.
Melzack, R. and Wall, P.D. Pain mechanisms: A new theory.
  Science, 1965, 150, 971-979.
Mitchell, J.F. Local anesthesia in general surgery. Jour-
  nal of the American Medical Association, 1907, 48, 198-
  201.
Notermans, S.L.H. Measurement of pain threshold determined
  by electrical stimulation and its clinical application.
  Part I. Methods and factors possible influencing the
  pain threshold. Neurology, 1966, 16, 1071-1086.
Price, H.L. and Dripps, R.D. Intravenous anesthetics. In
  The Pharmacological Basis of Therapeutics (Goodman, L.S.
  and Gilman, A., eds.). Fourth edition. New York: Macmillan, 1970, pp. 93-97.
Ratner, S.C. Comparative aspects of hypnosis. In Handbook
  of Clinical and Experimental Hypnosis. New York: Macmillan, 1967, pp. 550-587.
Reston, J. Now, about my operation. In Acupuncture: What
  Can It Do For You? New York: Newspaper Enterprise Assn.,
  1972, pp. 8-11.

Rhee, J.L. Introductory remarks: Acupuncture: The need
   for an in depth appraisal. In Transcript of the Acupuncture Symposium. Los Altos, Cal.: Academy of Parapsychology and Medicine, 1972, pp. 8-10.
Sampimon, R.L.N. and Woodruff, M.F.A. Some observations
   concerning the use of hypnosis as a substitute for anesthesia. Medical Journal of Australia, 1946, 1, 393-395.
Shealy, C.N. A physiological basis for electro-acupuncture.
   In Transcript of the Acupuncture Symposium. Los Altos,
   Cal.: Academy of Parapsychology and Medicine, 1972,
   pp. 34-36.
Shute, W.B. East meets West (1): Canadian eyes peek across
   the acupuncture threshold. Canadian Medical Association
   Journal, 1972, 107, 1002-1005.
Spanos, N.P., Barber, T.X., and Lang, G. Effects of hypnotic
   induction, suggestions of analgesia, and demands for
   honesty on subjective reports of pain. In Cognitive
   Alteration of Feeling States (London, H. and Nisbett, R.,
   eds.). Chicago: Aldine, in press.
Taub, T. Acupuncture. Science, 1972, 178, 9.
Tkach, W. A firsthand report from China: "I have seen acu-
   puncture work," says Nixon's doctor. Today's Health,
   1972, 50, (7) 50-56.
Toyama, P.M. and Nishizawa, M. The physiological basis of
   acupuncture therapy. North Carolina Medical Journal,
   1972, 33, 425-429.
Trent, J.C. Surgical anesthesia. Journal of the History
   of Medicine, 1946, 1, 505-511.
Tuckey, C.L. Psychotherapeutics: or treatment by hypnotism.
   Woods Medical and Surgical Monographs, 1889, 3, 721-795.
Veith, I. Acupuncture: Ancient enigma to East and West.
   American Journal of Psychiatry, 1972, 129, 333-336.
Wall, P. An eye on the needle. New Scientist, July 20,
   1972, pp. 129-131.
Warren, F.Z. Film presentation on acupuncture anesthesia.
   Panel discussion on acupuncture. In Transcript of the
   Acupuncture Symposium. Los Altos, Cal.: Academy of
   Parapsychology and Medicine, 1972, pp. 86-92.

A CLINICAL VIEW OF THE EFFECTIVENESS OF HYPNOSIS IN PAIN CONTROL

Kay F. Thompson

University of Pittsburgh School of Dental
Medicine
Pittsburgh, Pennsylvania

Hypnosis can be a useful tool in the control of many types of pain, if the practitioner first understands something of the dynamics of hypnosis. A lack of knowledge about the clinical hypnotic situation has been partially responsible for the delay in the acceptance of the professional use of hypnosis as a treatment for many problems regarding pain. It is a difficult subject to study scientifically because the hypnotic situation is not a constant It fluctuates with the needs of both the patient and the doctor. In treatment of pain, hypnosis, like aspirin, may not be appropriate or effective for many patients. It is, however, "one of the possible approaches to the handling of the patient's problems that possesses special and highly significant values at both the psychological and physiological levels."[1]

There are many interpretations of hypnosis, partly because there are so many facets to it. The concept of hypnosis which for years has been fostered by the stage hypnotist is one of zombie-like unconsciousness where the person in a trance must follow the commands of the hypnotist. This is a fascinating but offensive concept which has been demonstrated to be inaccurate. The concept of hypnosis as a state of hyperacuity and heightened control which may occur spontaneously in any stress situation may be uncomfortable, too. It means that hypnosis may occur in any interpersonal situation and infers that the doctor should be aware of this possibility. The most easily accepted idea is that hypnosis is simply an altered state of consciousness. If we accept the idea that in this

altered state of consciousness, there can be an increased
capacity to accept suggestions, then it can be understood
that in the hypnotic trance the patient can respond to helpful suggestions from the doctor which might otherwise be
disregarded.

One thing which can be said in favor of hypnosis that
cannot be said for most other approaches to treatment of
pain is that it cannot do any damage to the patient. The
worst thing that can happen is that nothing happens! The
doctor, then, is just where he would have been if hypnosis
had not been attempted. There have been no drugs, medications or treatments for the pain which might act adversely.

Hypnosis does offer one method of making a situation
more tolerable for the patient who is frightened of pain.
Part of the fear of pain can be the fear of behaving poorly,
of making a fool of oneself over pain. Another part is
fear of the unknown, and of the loss of control.[2] Finally,
there is the fear of the pain itself. The patient can
learn to utilize the trance state to handle any or all
parts of the potentially painful situation with reasonable
comfort and dignity. Pain has its physical and psychosomatic aspects. Hypnosis is an effective method for treating the psychosomatic aspects and minimizing the physical
ones, where everything is being done to treat the cause of
the pain.

There are those who believe that the only thing hypnosis
does is to teach the patient to relax. Even if this were
true, it would still be a valuable tool, since this hypnotic
technique utilizes the scientifically proven relationship
that with a decrease in tension there is an increased pain
threshold. The person who comes to the professional appointment uptight and frightened, tense and apprehensive,
can learn to concentrate and relax, and go into a useful
trance state in which the tolerance level and pain threshold are both increased. Clinicians generally acknowledge
that a relaxed patient is more comfortable and cooperative,
as a result of which the doctor is also more relaxed and
better able to do the best possible job for the patient.

Current approaches to pain must consider the subjective viewpoint of the patient, since it is, after all, "his"
pain. At a hypnosis workshop Ernest Hilgard, Ph.D.,[3]

elaborated on the idea of "pain" versus "suffering", and
said that the pain which comes before the injury can cause
as much or more suffering than the actual trauma. "Anticipation" is a popular pastime for individuals about to undergo the introduction of pain into their lives. In this
situation it makes little difference where the pain is,
where it comes from, or what kind it is. The patient may
require help to stop it. One of my patients taught me a
lesson about pain, when she requested the assistance of
hypnosis during the extraction of four bone-impacted third
molars. When I tried to persuade her to visit an oral
surgeon and have a general anesthetic for the operation,
she said, "I know you can take care of the physical pain,
it is the psychological pain I am concerned about." She
learned hypnosis well, and the teeth were removed with local
anesthesia and hypnosis. Recovery was rapid and uneventful,
with no swelling or discoloration, uninterrupted by any
post-operative pain.

Pain can be relatively easy for the doctor to control
until there is a need to determine what value the patient
places on the pain and/or the suffering. The question then
becomes how to determine the value system, if the pain is
to be approached hypnotically or otherwise. The perception
of the pain stimulus is a response to:

1. physical injury
2. psychological injury
3. both
4. anticipation of either.

The control of pain is affected by many factors, which include:

1. social: learned, cultural response, as when a
   child falls and is "hurt", but cries only when
   there is someone there to respond to the crying;
2. physical: immobilization of a fracture, surgery;
3. physiological/pharmacological: medication, anti-
   biotics, sedatives;
4. psychological: reassurance, hypnosis, psychotherapy.

Hypnosis is not a substitute for any other appropriate
actions which should be taken in determination and diagnosis
of pain. All possible medical, surgical and therapeutic

procedures should be followed in addition to the introduction of hypnosis. It does not reduce the responsibility of
the doctor, but it enhances the effectiveness of treatment,
and enables the patient to cooperate more completely. Once
the phenomena of the pain, acute or chronic, has been investigated thoroughly, it may be determined whether hypnosis
could be helpful.

Indications for the use of hypnosis in the control and
relief of pain rely on a variety of factors, dependent primarily on the "kind" of pain and the "kind" of patient. As
Dr. Leonard Monheim, Professor of Anesthesia,[4] taught,
"When you understand the patient, you've gone a long way
toward understanding the pain." Hypnosis enables the patient to restructure his attitude toward, need for, and
satisfaction from pain. He learns to reduce his response
of tension and anxiety and inhibit the usual autonomic
nervous system reactions to perception of painful stimuli.
It should be remembered that it is the result of what the
patient does in the hypnotic state, rather than the induction of it, that provides the change and the potential pain
relief. When the doctor teaches the patient how to enter
the hypnotic state, this does nothing other than introduce
the possibility that changes can occur. Ability to utilize
the trance state requires patient motivation for pain relief, and some level of understanding that this relief is
possible.

One possible approach which might be utilized clinically is one which has been effective with my patients. It
is a very simple explanation about pain, but one which can
be understood in a number of ways. The patient is first
taught to go into a trance, either with the usual relaxation
techniques or with ones utilizing tension and focusing on
pain. While in the trance, the patient is told, "Pain is
a danger or a warning signal. When the reason for the pain
is known and understood, and everything that can and should
be done for the pain has been done, then there is no longer
any reason to suffer from pain." For posthypnotic post-
surgical pain relief, the suggestion is included that, "You
can be pleasantly surprised to learn how comfortable you
can be as long as normal healing is progressing."

This oversimplified rationale expects the following
"understandings" by the patient. The first statement is

that pain is a necessary stimulus to alert him that something is happening to which he should pay attention, and take appropriate action. The second concept involves the need to learn what has happened, and to know that all appropriate action has been taken. This does not imply that the patient is well, or even that he will get better. "Everything that can be done..." also infers that it is possible that enough cannot be done for him to recover, but that he can learn to maintain a degree of comfort required to function satisfactorily with his illness. This approach is useful with chronic pain, and in terminal cases such as maligancies, since it gives the patient permission to control or eliminate the pain to the degree desired. The posthypnotic suggestion for recovery from surgery does not say that there will be no pain, since that determination is up to the patient. It includes again the idea of a degree of comfort acceptable to the patient. There is also the suggestion that if normal healing is not occurring there will be pain, and this statement is based on the general agreement that clinical patients have not been able, with hypnosis, to mask pain in order to ignore it, and avoid seeking appropriate medical assistance. If the pain is purely an affective emotional response the patient can also be offered the help of hypnosis to "let go" of the pain, much as the hysterical child, who cries when the reason for the crying has long since passed, can be interrupted and distracted. The patient can accept a semi-logical rationale as a mechanism to interrupt the cycle of expectation of pain.

The control of the autonomic nervous system that is made possible through hypnosis can enhance the relief of pain, utilizing semi-logical rationale for suggestions. The patient can be told either, "Pain interferes with healing," or, "Pain stimulates healing." With the "Pain interferes with healing" rationale, the awareness of the pain demands the expenditure of energy to combat the pain, with its tension, inflammation, swelling, congestion, and physical discomfort. All these symptoms distract from and delay the healing process. With the "Pain stimulates healing" rationale, the signals from the injured area carry the message for increased circulation, which encourages the blood stream to carry the healing nutrients more rapidly to that area, and to carry away the cells responsible for the

inflammatory, congested response resulting in pain. The
healing process can proceed rapidly, without interruption
by pain. Either verbalization can be successful in treating patients who are highly motivated to get rid of or
control their pain.

All of my discussion is relative to clinical pain, and
is based on the internal motivation of the patient. Motivation, I feel, is the principle difference between clinical and experimental findings on hypnosis and pain. In the
clinical trance the learning comes from internal motivation,
with the trance a selfish one. This is particularly true
once the patient recognizes that his pain is real, and there
is no way to back out. The clinical pain belongs to the
patient and originates inside him, and this knowledge can
be utilized in his trance to help himself. In the experimental situation the subject volunteers to participate in
an experiment, and the forms he signs specify the limitations involved. The pain originates from an external stimulus, while the subject retains the option to back out any
time. The motivation is more externally directed, for
"science, mankind and money". This type of experimental
research is significant, as long as the differences in
motivational criteria are recognized.

The variety of needs for pain relief are as diverse
and interrelated as their causes. Hypnosis, appropriately
taught to patients, is a valuable adjunct to other methods
of pain relief. It may provide the fastest method of treating the psychosomatic aspects of pain, and in many cases is
better than chemotherapy for treating the physical aspects.
In the least effective case hypnosis relaxes the patient,
and in the best case it permits the patient to control his
pain once he understands it.

REFERENCES

1. Haley, Jay, editor: Advanced techniques of hypnosis
      and therapy: selected papers of Milton H. Erickson,
      M.D., New York, Grune and Stratton, 1967, p. 435.
2. Mowrer, O.H. and Viek, P.: An experimental analogue
      of fear from a sense of helplessness, in McClelland,
      D.C.: Studies in motivation, New York, Appleton-
      Crofts, 1955.

3. Hilgard, E.R.,San Francisco, July, 1974.
4. Monheim, L.M., University of Pittsburgh School of Dental
        Medicine, Lecture, Emergencies in the dental office,
        1961.

PSYCHOPHYSIOLOGICAL RATIONALE FOR THE APPLICATION OF

BIOFEEDBACK IN THE ALLEVIATION OF PAIN

Charles F. Stroebel and Bernard C. Glueck

Institute of Living

Hartford, Connecticut

By elucidating the apparent psychophysiologic mechanisms affected by biofeedback in the treatment of psychosomatic conditions, considerable qualification must be extended to sweeping claims currently being made for the application of this new treatment modality to the problem of pain. This discussion will conclude that biofeedback is largely ineffective after the onset of the sensation of pain, except in reducing the level of activation of the emergency fight or flight response and in reducing muscular "bracing against" the pain. However, clinical experience does indicate that biofeedback can be highly effective in a preventive sense, altering physiology so that the antecedent mechanisms leading to the production of pain do not occur. The psychophysiologic mechanisms presumed to be operating in muscular contraction and vascular headache pain will be used as illustrative, since experience in treating these conditions with biofeedback is most extensive at the present time.

In contrast to our conscious awareness of the five senses and the extensive kinesthetic-position feedback from the striate musculature, functional reporting at the conscious level from smooth muscles, glands, and the gamma efferent regulation of striate muscle tension is meager, except under conditions of malfunction. The major sensation with malfunction of the latter systems is the relatively crude sensation of pain, sometimes referred to a distant dermatome. In other words, we are relatively unaware of blood pressure, of gastrointestinal peristaltic activity, of cardiac mechanics, of vasomotor regulation—the "involuntary"

inner machinery of the body--except when significant malfunction occurs. While the adaptive regulation of inner machinery under conditions of normalcy indicates that reporting is
largely at an unconscious level, probably not ascending
above the limbic system and is not normally under "voluntary"
control.

The basic psychophysiologic principle of biofeedback is
in providing parallel proprioception, via an external biofeedback loop, so that an inner machinery function becomes
observable at the conscious level. This is accomplished with
suitable sensors (electrical, thermal, pressure, etc.), electronics, and audio, visual, or tactile feedback signals. Considerable experimental controversy currently exists as to how
animals and man use this parallel proprioception to gain voluntary control of the inner machinery function in question
(e.g., operant conditioning, mediation, suggestion, placebo
effect, etc.) (Stroebel and Glueck, 1973). However, voluntary control has now been demonstrated for many physiological
systems under relatively passive learning conditions (i.e.,
voluntary control is difficult to demonstrate if the subject
"tries too hard"). Noteworthy is the fact that for most patients who have begun to experience a pain sensation their motivation is anything but "passive." Further, the pain stimulus apparently serves as a significant distraction to the
mental processes evoked in achieving voluntary regulation.

Two major clinical applications of biofeedback which are
becoming increasingly widespread, even in traditional headache clinics, are alterations of antecedent mechanisms of
muscular contractions (tenstion) headaches and of vascular
(migraine) headaches.

In 1970 Budzynski, Stoyva and Adler reported a significant reduction in the severity and frequency of muscle con-
striction headaches when patients learned voluntary reduction
of EMG frontalis tension via EMG biofeedback. While the contraction of striate muscle is under voluntary control, voluntary reduction of tension in individuals predisposed to tension headaches apparently is not. The underlying physiologic
mechanism is probably a faulty homeostatic "oversetting" of
the gamma efferent system which regulates striate muscles so
as to always be prepared to produce movement without "slack."
Through biofeedback these patients reacquire the ability to
not overset (or "over brace") the gamma efferent regulatory
system.

Several lines of evidence suggest that the actual pain of the tension headache results from local reflexive spasm ("cramp") of striate muscle from prolonged unconsicous bracing and fatigue. Once local spasm and pain begin, central nervous system control, such as would be exerted via biofeedback training, becomes largely ineffective. In a series of 42 tension headache patinets receiving biofeedback EMG frontalis training at the Institute of Living only two could utilize biofeedback to abort the headache once it began. However, 38 of the 42 reported significant reduction in severity and frequency and significant reduction in usage of analgesics six months after learning voluntary EMG reduction. These results may be summarized to suggest that regular practice of biofeedback acquired EMG reduction had apparent prophylactic value, but little effect in the event of a "breakthrough" headache occurring.

In 1973 Sargent, Walters and Green reported significant reduction in frequency of vascular (migraine) headache in 80% of patients receiving thermal feedback to differentially warm their hands and "cool" their foreheads (slight forehead warming actually occurs). This result, confirmed clinically in several centers, has unfortunately created a misunderstanding about the potentials of biofeedback in the treatment of pain after its onset. The differential technique of forehead cooling and handwarming implied a similarity in the mechanism of thermal biofeedback and a commonly used migraine medication (caffeine and ergotamine), namely vasoconstriction (i.e., reduced blood flow and cooling) of extracranial arteries. In a series of 91 vascular headache patients treated with thermal biofeedback at the Institute of Living, no single patient could abort the headache once pain onset had occurred, whereas most received some relief from cafergot. On the other hand, 30 out of 31 of the classical migraine patients (i.e., clear vasoconstrictive prodrome, such as a scintillating scotoma or blurred vision) could prevent pain onset one month after biofeedback training if they performed handwarming (vasodilation) as soon as the prodrome symptoms appeared. Measurements revealed that modest forehead warming, not cooling, was associated with handwarming skill.

In contrast, only three out of the 60 common migraine patients (no vasoconstrictive prodrome before the pain onset) reported reduced headache frequency at one month; this figure rose to 32 out of 60 after six months after prolonged generalization practice of handwarming for several minutes during every waking hour. Even for this success group, their biofeedback technique was ineffective after onset of pain in a breakthrough headache.

The following mechanism for biofeedback treatment of vascular headache can be advanced to explain these perplexing results. In the classical form the vascular headache begins with vasoconstriction of extracranial cerebral arteries via sympathetic outflow, potentially compromising cerebral and retinal circulation and producing the vasoconstrictive prodromal symptoms. As potential ischemia becomes impending, a protective "fuse" chemical, designated as a neurokinin, is released in the walls of the vessels, metabolically blocking sympathetic activation of arterial smooth muscle, permitting reflexive engorgement of the vessels and stretching of arterial wall pain receptors, thus producing the migraine headache pain.

The mechanism of thermal biofeedback is an apparent prophylactic one of preventing the extreme degree of sympathetic nervous system induced vasoconstriction and ischemia which triggers regression to local release of neurokinin. Once this local release has occurred, decreases or increases in sympathetic activation achieved via biofeedback are ineffective, while medications with a direct myotonic mechanism (i.e., arterial muscle constrictors such as ergotamine tartrate) remain somewhat effective. Duration of the migraine pain, which is often quite consistent for a specific patient, is apparently related to the time required for reestablishing sympathetic nervous control of arterial smooth muscle (i.e., reversal of the metabolic blockage of the nerve-muscle interface).

Classic migraine patients are, in a sense fortunate, since the prodromal period gives them a brief opportunity to use biofeedback exercises to lessen the sympathetic outflow and vasoconstriction which would lead to the local events producing the headache pain. Common migraine patients, however, begin to experience reduced headache frequency only after they have acquired a general tendency, 24 hours a day, to reduce sympathetic outflow and vasoconstriction. Using the biofeedback treatment protocol adopted at the Institute of Living, four to six months of biofeedback training and self practice are needed to achieve a sufficient degree of generalization for common migraine sufferers.

Neither classic nor common migraine patients in our series have found biofeedback effective once pain (reflex engorgement) begins. Common migraine patients find this particularly depressing as they continue to experience breakthrough headaches during their four to six month training period. This failure to obtain immediate symptom relief may be advanced as one rationale for the difference in improvement rates between classic and common diagnostic categories.

Noteworthy is the fact that no single patient in our series has been able to effect significant EMG frontalis tension reduction or vasodilation (handwarming) while they are actually experiencing pain. Hence patients must be pain free to acquire biofeedback skills, a serious limiting factor in application of biofeedback to chornic pain problems.

If voluntary vasodilation of overly constricted cephalic arteries is the prophylactic mechanism of biofeedback in vascular headache, it would seem efficacious to teach head warming directly. Why teach handwarming at all? Definitive data do not yet exist to resolve this issue, but preliminary evidence indicates that acquisition of handwarming, with subsequent generalization through imagery to cephalic vessels, occurs more rapidly than direct cephalic training.

In summary, the mechanisms of EMG frontalis tension reduction and vasodilation (thermal) biofeedback apparently operate via central nervous system mechanisms and are effective prophylactically in preventing pain onset unless protective regression to local reflexive action takes place. Once local reflexive spasm or chemical inhibition of muscle-nerve interfaces and associated sensations of pain occur, biofeedback is largely ineffective. The presence of pain per se makes acquisition of voluntary regulation of smooth and striate muscle tension exceedingly difficult, particularly when reflexive local mechanisms limit the possible effect of central nervous system intervention. Any of a variety of general relaxation techniques, as listed in Figure 1, are probably equivalent to biofeedback training in reducing the contribution of the activation level of the

GENERAL

OBJECTIVES:

1) RELAXATION

2) LOWERING OF TENSION

3) STATES INCOMPATIBLE WITH EMERGENCY FIGHT OR FLIGHT RESPONSE

EEG ALPHA

EEG THETA

FRONTALIS EMG

NON BIOFEEDBACK MODALITIES

PASSIVE MEDITATION

BENSON RELAXATION RESPONSE

AUTOGENIC TRAINING

PROGRESSIVE RELAXATION

SPECIFIC

OBJECTIVES:

1) TO REGULATE OR LOWER THE ACTIVATION OF A TARGET ORGAN SYMPTOM

THERMAL (SMOOTH MUSCLE RELAXATION)

CLASSIC MIGRAINE – VASCULAR HEADACHE (RAPID)

COMMON MIGRAINE – VASCULAR HEADACHE (SLOW)

RAYNAUD'S DISEASE

IRRITABLE COLON SYNDROME

ESSENTIAL HYPERTENSION

ANGINA PECTORIS

FRONTALIS EMG

TENSION – MUSCULAR CONTRACTION HEADACHE

BRUXISM

TMJ SYNDROME

LUMBAR-SACRAL EMG

MUSCULAR BACK PAIN

EKG

CARDIAC DYSRHYTHMIAS

GSR AND THERMAL

HYPERTENSION

STRESS ASPECT OF ECZEMATOUS CONDITIONS

Fig. 1. Applications of Biofeedback

fight or flight emergency response or bracing maneuvers which exacerbate the sensation of pain (Glueck and Stroebel, 1975).

REFERENCES

1. Budzynski, T.H., Stoyva, J.M., and Adler, C.S.: Feedback-induced muscle relaxation: Application to tension headache, Behav. Ther. Exp. Psychiatry, 1:205–211, 1970.

2. Glueck, B.C., and Stroebel, C.F.: Biofeedback and meditation in the treatment of psychiatric Illnesses, Compr. Psychiatry, 16:303–321, 1975.

3. Sargent, J.D., Walters, E.D., and Green, E.E.: Psychosomatic self regulation of migraine headaches, Sem. in Psychiatry, 3:416–428, 1973.

4. Stroebel, C.F., and Glueck, B.C.: Biofeedback treatment in medicine and psychiatry, In Birk, L.(ed.) Biofeedback: Behavioral Medicine, New York, Grune and Stratton, 1973.

LONG-TERM EVALUATION OF CONSERVATIVE TREATMENT FOR

MYOFASCIAL PAIN-DYSFUNCTION SYNDROME

Charles S. Greene and Daniel M. Laskin

University of Illinois College of Dentistry

Chicago, Illinois

The treatment of any disorder is based on two fundamental considerations: the pathophysiology of the condition
and its cause or causes. There currently is rather broad
agreement that masticatory muscle fatigue and spasm are responsible for the cardinal symptoms of pain, tenderness,
clicking, and limited function that characterize the myofascial pain-dysfunction (MPD) syndrome.[1-3] The question
of cause, however, has remained controversial, and as a result, treatment of the MPD syndrome has varied accordingly.

At this time, the most widely accepted hypothesis for
the origin of MPD problems is based on the assumption that
various types of so-called occlusal disharmonies can disrupt
normal neuromuscular function, and that in certain individuals this situation can lead to muscular fatigue and
spasm.[4-6] Clinicians who subscribe to this hypothesis spend
a good deal of time observing, recording, and analyzing
occlusal relationships when they examine patients with MPD.
Then, in the treatment phase, these clinicians believe it
is necessary to correct the occlusal disharmonies to "eliminate the cause." The extent of the occlusal correction
can vary from equilibration[3-5,7] to full-mouth reconstruc-
tion,[5,8,9] and may also include bite opening,[10,11] ortho-
dontic treatment,[12] or both.

Extensive research conducted during the past 10 to 15

From the Journal of the American Dental Association 89:1365-
1368, Copyright 1974, American Dental Association. Reprinted
by permission.

years, however, has led other investigators to conclude that
the muscular fatigue and spasm in most patients with MPD is
caused primarily by emotional stress rather than by mechanical factors, and they have proposed the psychophysiologic
theory for MPD origin.[13-16] Those who subscribe to this
theory have reported success in the treatment of MPD with
various conservative modalities such as medications,[17]
splints,[18] and psychological counseling,[19,20] but without
making alterations of occlusion.

     Most clinicians acknowledge that such conservative treat-
ment can be helpful to patients with MPD. However, proponents of occlusal disharmony theories assume that this type
of treatment merely provides temporary symptomatic relief,
which must be accompanied or followed by definitive occlusal
correction. Several longitudinal studies have shown that
most patients with MPD who are treated successfully with oc-
clusion-modifying techniques continue to do well as long as
a few years later,[21-24] but no one has reported previously
on the long-term effects of the more conservative treatment
approaches. This paper reports the long-term status of a
large series of patients with MPD who were treated during the
past ten years with a variety of conservative modalities.

STUDY METHOD

     Participants in this study were 135 patients with
chronic MPD syndrome who had been treated at the Temporomandibular Joint Research Center, University of Illinois,
until they were dismissed after either successfully or unsuccessfully completing treatment. Intervals of six months
to eight years, with an average interval of three years,
had elapsed since these individuals were dismissed. Patients
who failed to complete treatment were not included in this
study, nor were those who were found to have organic disorders of the temporomandibular joint.

     The treatment modalities that were used for the patients
varied over the years as different clinical studes were
conducted. They included such conservative and reversible
modalities as analgesics, tranquilizers, exercises, splints,
joint and muscle injections, physical therapy, psychological
counseling, and placebos. The results of these studies have
been described in previous papers.[17-20,25-30] Regardless

of the therapy used, treatment was always accompanied by a
combination of reassurance, explanation, advice for self-
management, and a general attitude of sympathetic understanding. The patients routinely were tested and inter-
viewed by staff psychologists, and the relationship between
emotional stress, oral habits, muscle tension, and MPD symptoms was emphasized repeatedly throughout their clinical
appointments.

On their dismissal, all patients were advised to obtain
routine dental care as needed. For certain patients, this
included crowns, fixed bridgework, partial dentures, or even
complete dentures. Although some of these dental restora-
tions may have produced changes in occlusal relationships,
patients were never advised specifically to have equilibration, bite-opening, or major reconstructive procedures. In
fact, they generally were advised to avoid these types of
treatment. Therefore, the great majority of patients in
this study did not have any irreversible modifications of
occlusal relationships either during or after treatment of
their MPD problems.

The follow-up survey of patients with MPD who were
treated at the center was started in 1971, when a recall
system was initiated. A standardized questionnaire was designed for telephone interview of patients who could not
come in for direct obervation. With the use of several
hundred clinical records, lists were made of successfully
and unsuccessfully treated patients. Since patients who
did not complete the recommended course of treatment were
not included in this study, the list if unsuccessfully
treated patients was rather small. An attempt was made to
contact all of these patients, and eventually a sample of
35 was obtained. By comparison, the list of successfully
treated patients included several hundred names from which
a random sample was collected until the arbitrary number of
100 was attained. Thus, 135 patients were either seen at
the center or contacted by telephone to obtain the data for
this study.

The successfully treated patients were asked how they
were feeling currently, whether they had any recurrent MPD
symptoms since being dismissed, how they were able to manage these symptoms if they did occur, and whether any further professional treatment had been needed for their MPD

problems. The unsuccessfully treated patients were asked
how they were feeling currently, whether they had sought
further professional treatment after leaving the center,
and whether such treatment had been helpful for them.

RESULTS

The survey of the long-term status of the 100 successfully treated patients at the center showed that more than
half (51) reported that they were functioning very well and
feeling quite comfortable, with no episodes of recurrent
MPD symptoms since completing treatment. Forty-one patients
reported that they also were doing quite well, but had occasional minor episodes of pain, dysfunction, or both, which
they could manage adequately through the use of voluntary
relaxation techniques, medications, or exercises. Two patients had experienced a major episode of recurrent MPD symptoms within a few months after leaving the center. They
returned for treatment which then provided long-term relief.
Only 6 of the 100 patients reported that their MPD problems
were not under control since they had left the center.

After the data were collected for the 35 unsuccessfully
treated patients, they were separated into two subgroups:
those patients who sought further professional treatment
and those who did not. The long-term status of the patients
in these two subgroups is summarized in the Table. The 15
patients who had sought further professional help received
a variety of treatments including equilibration, bite opening, extractions, joint and muscle injections, and surgery.
The other 20 patients either continued wearing splints or
doing exercises at home, or they simply stopped treatment
altogether.

Regardless of whether they had received subsequent
professional attention for MPD symptoms, the condition of
nearly half of the 35 unsuccessfully treated patients improved within several months or years after leaving the
center, whereas the condition of the others did not. No
one particular treatment was found to be especially effective for those patients who were treated successfully by
other practitioners.

TABLE = Long-term status of 35 unsuccessfully treated
patients with MPD.

| | Improved | | Not Improved | |
	Totally	Partially	No change	Worse
Patients who received subsequent professional treatment (N=15)	2	4(40%)	8	1(60%)
Patients who did not receive subsequent professional treatment (N=20)	4	5(45%)	8	3(55%)

DISCUSSION

The results obtained in this study of conservatively
treated patients with MPD indicate that those individuals
who respond favorably to such treatment generally will continue to feel comfortable and function well over long periods
of time. This is true regardless of which particular treatment they received and even regardless of whether the treatment was "real" or placebo. However, this study also indicates that a patient who had an unfavorable response to
conservative therapy has about the same chance of eventually
improving or staying the same, regardless of whether he receives more aggressive physical treatment or does nothing
at all.

Comparison of our results with those reported previously
for occlusally treated patients[21-24] shows no significant
difference between the long-term success rates of these diverse treatment approaches. Therefore, one can conclude
that in a psychophysiologic disorder such as MPD syndrome,
the most important factor in successful management does not
depend on the specific treatment used but rather on the
general approach to the patient. The establishment of a
good dentist-patient rapport and explanation of the nature
of the problem appear to be of primary importance. This

conclusion is supported by the results of Lupton's study of the effectiveness of psychological counseling and cognitive programs in the treatment of patients with MPD.[20]

For nonresponding patients with MPD, the same principles apply in reverse. In general, their failure to respond does not seem to be attributable to insufficient or incorrect physical forms of therapy, but rather to complex psychological factors that interfere with the dentist-patient relationship. R. Schwartz[31] in a comparison of the Minnesota Multiphasic Personality Inventory scores of responsive and nonresponsive patients with MPD, found a much greater amount of psychopathology in the latter group. Moreover, Pomp has shown that many patients with MPD who do not improve with conventional treatment of any kind do respond well to short-term psychotherapy.[19] Similar conclusions have been reported in connection with other functional psychophysiologic disorders.[32,33]

Since this study shows that the specific physical form of therapy does not seem to be the essential factor in the determination of long-term success or failure in treatment of patients with MPD, it seems logical to use the most conservative modalities in combination with supportive communication techniques and to avoid over-treatment with radical or complex modalities. Moreover, any attempt by clinicians to characterize treatments for the MPD syndrome as either symptom-relieving or definitive seems to be meaningless. Instead, in a population of patients who respond positively to so many different treatments, a more useful distinction can be made between conservative and radical, between appropriate and inappropriate, or between adequate and excessive treatment.

REFERENCES

1. Perry, H.T., Jr. The symptomology of temporomandibular joint disturbance. J Prosthet Dent 19:288, March 1968.

This investigation was supported by USPHS Grant DE-02899.

The authors thank Dr. Charles F. Lockhart for his help in collection of the data.

2. Franks, A.S.   Masticatory muscle hyperactivity and tem-
    poromandibular joint dysfunction. J Prosthet Dent
    15:112 Nov-Dec 1965.
3. Ramfjord, S.P.   Dysfunctional temporomandibular joint
    and muscle pain. J Prosthet Dent 11:353 March-April
    1961.
4. Krogh-Poulsen, W.G., and Olsson, A.   Occlusal dishar-
    monies and dysfunction of the stomatognathic system.
    Dent Clin North Am 10:627 Nov 1966.
5. Ramfjord, S.P., and Ash, M.M. Occlusion. Philadelphia,
    W. B. Saunders Co., 1966, chapter 8.
6. Shore, N.A.   Occlusal equilibration and temporomandibular
    joint dysfunction. Philadelphia, J. B. Lippincott
    Co., 1959, chapter 6.
7. Jankelson, B.   Technique for obtaining optimum function-
    al relationship for the natural dentition. Dent Clin
    North Am March 1960, p. 131.
8. Mann, A.W., and Pankey, L.D. Concepts of occlusion: the
    PM philosophy of occlusal rehabilitation. Dent Clin
    North Am Nov 1963, p 621.
9. Posselt, U.O.A.   Physiology of occlusion and rehabilita-
    tion, ed 2. Philadelphia, F. A. Davis Co., 1968,
    chapter 7.
10. Graber, T.M.   Overbite-the dentist's challenge. JADA
    79:1135 Nov 1969.
11. Block, L.S.   Diagnosis and treatment of disturbances of
    the temporomandibular joint especially in relation
    to vertical dimension. JADA 34:253 Feb 15, 1947.
12. Salzmann, J.A.   Practice of orthodontics. Philadelphia,
    J. B. Lippincott Co., 1966, p 572.
13. Schwartz, L., and others.   Disorders of the temporoman-
    dibular joint, diagnosis, management, relation to
    occlusion of teeth. Philadelphia, W. B. Saunders
    Co., 1959, chapter 2.
14. Moulton, R.E.   Emotional factors in non-organic temporo-
    mandibular joint pain. Dent Clin North Am Nov 1966,
    p 609.
15. Lupton, D.E.   Psychological aspects of temporomandibular
    joint dysfunction. JADA 79:131 July 1969.
16. Laskin, D.M.   Etiology of the pain-dysfunction syndrome.
    JADA 79:147 July 1969.
17. Greene, C.S., and Laskin, D.M.   Meprobamate therapy for
    the myofascial pain-dysfunction (MPD) syndome: a
    double-blind evaluation. JADA 82:587 March 1971.

18. Greene, C.S., and Laskin, D.M. Splint therapy for the
     myofascial pain-dysfunction (MPD) syndrome: a com-
     parative study. JADA 84:624 March 1972.
19. Pomp, A.M. Psychotherapy for the myofascial pain-dys-
     function (MPD) syndrome: a study of factors coin-
     ciding with symptom remission. JADA 89:629 Sept
     1974.
20. Lupton, D.E. A comparative analysis of the effective-
     ness of counseling, instruction, and dental treat-
     ment, thesis. University of Chicago, Chicago, 1967.
21. Dachi, S.F. Diagnosis and management of temporomandi-
     bular joint dysfunction syndrome. J Prosthet Dent
     20:53 July 1968.
22. Zarb, G.A., and Thompson, G.W. Assessment of clinical
     treatment of patients with temporomandibular joint
     dysfunction. J Prosthet Dent 24:542 Nov 1970.
23. Carraro, J.J., Caffesse, R.G., and Albano, E.A. Temporo-
     mandibular joint syndrome—a clinical evaluation.
     Oral Surg 28:54 July 1969.
24. Posselt, U. The temporomandibular joint syndrome and
     occlusion. J Prosthet Dent 25:432 April 1971.
25. Lerman, M.D. A preliminary study of muscle exercises
     in treatment of the TMJ pain-dysfunction syndrome.
     Abstracted, IADR Program & Abstracts no. 564 March
     1968.
26. Shipman, W.G., Greene, C.S., and Laskin, D.M. Correla-
     tion of placebo responses and personality character-
     istics in myofascial pain-dysfunction (MPD) patients.
     J Psychosom Res. to be published.
27. Greene, C.S., and Laskin, D.M. Correlation of placebo
     responses and psychological characteristics in myo-
     fascial pain-dysfunction (MPD) patinets. Abstracted,
     IADR Program & Abstracts no. 282 March 1970.
28. Greene, C.S., and Laskin, D.M. Therapeutic effects of
     diazepam (Valium) and sodium salicylate in myofas-
     cial pain-dysfunction (MPD) patients. Abstracted,
     IADR Program & Abstracts no. 193 March 1972.
29. Laskin, D.M., and Greene, C.S. Influence of the doctor-
     patient relationship on placebo therapy for patients
     with myofascial pain-dysfunction (MPD) syndrome.
     JADA 85:892 Oct 1972.
30. Goodman, P., and Greene, C.S. Response to placebo
     equilibration in MPD patients. J Dent Res 52 (special
     issue): 76, abstract no. 72 Feb 1973.

31. Schwartz, R.A. Personality characteristics of unsuccessfully treated MPD patients. J Dent Res 53 (special issue): 127, abstract no. 291 Feb 1974.
32. Sternbach, R.A., and others. Aspects of chronic low-back pain. Psychosomatics 14:52 Jan-Feb 1973.
33. Sternbach, R.A., and others. Traits of pain patients: the low-back "loser". Read before 19th annual meeting of Academy of Psychosomatic Medicine, San Diego, Calif, Oct 29-Nov 1, 1972.

PAIN CONTROL AS A FACTOR IN PREVENTIVE HEALTH CARE

Jeannette F. Rayner

U. S. Public Health Service

Bethesda, Maryland

An extensive literature on preventive health behavior
provides ample documentation of the multiple factors functioning on the cultural, social, and psychological level for
individuals who seek preventive care. Kegeles (1963), Rosenstock (1969), Gochman (1971), Green(1970), Newman and Anderson (1972), Lambert and Freeman (1965), Weisenberg (1973),
O'Shea and Gray (1968), Hochbaum (1959), and Mechanic (1968)
are only a few of those who have specified factors which
prompt the seeking of care for preventive reasons. Kegeles,
Hochbaum, Rosenstock, and Gochman have identified relevant
psychological variables. Green, O'Shea and Gray, Mechanic,
Lambert and Freeman, and Newman and Anderson have examined
the sociological dimensions. Yet a more accurate statement
is that virtually all studies have transcended disciplines
and each has in either greater or lesser degree, dealt with
socio-psychological combinations of factors and their interactions. Cultural factors in respect to preventive behaviors have received less attention. At least there seems to
have been less effort expended toward explaining preventive
health behavior as specific cultural norms. Rather responses to medical or dental care or the onset of symptoms
are studied as expressions of cultural orientations. Zola
(1966), Hetherington and Harper (1962), and Zborowski
(1969) are among those who typify this approach. Zola, however, points out the importance of cultural influences in
preventive medicine and public health. Pettibone and Solis
(1973) studied dental care in cultural groups of the American southwest. Symptomatic and preventive orientations were
among the variables studied.

There is also an equally extensive literature on various aspects of pain, e.g., pain thresholds, pain tolerance, and psychogenic effects of pain. But the role of social and cultural factors in pain as <u>deterents</u> to care is less well documented. Zborowski and the others mentioned above, deal with cultural aspects of the definition and behavioral responses to pain which suggests that pain and the fear of pain may operate to delay seeking treatment.

The purpose of this paper is that of reviewing whatever information is available on the role of pain and its relationship to preventive health behavior. Emphasis will be on pain as a factor in preventive <u>dental</u> health behavior, for it is in respect to dental care that pain is most commonly assumed to be a deterent to seeking care. More accurately, it is <u>assumed</u> that <u>fear</u> of pain is the anti-motivator.

Fourteen years ago, Cole (1961) stated that dentistry had failed to give adequate consideration to the factors which deter patients from seeking the care they need. Of the 500 persons responding to his questionnaire, 20% indicated fear of pain as the reason for not seeking care-- and this is for <u>known needed</u> care. Thirty-four percent admitted being afraid of pain before <u>every</u> dental visit.

Thomas (1965) surveyed a college population in 1965 and found that "equal numbers fear the dentist as don't."

More recently, Richardson (1972) reviewed the role of fear as a dental problem. He states that "twelve million people avoid dental treatment because of fear" and further, that "pain and fear have been so closely associated with dentistry that patients have considered the terms synonymous."

Beecher (1959) on the psychogenics of pain states that "the pain experience is related not only to the intensity of the noxious stimulus but also to the threat value of the stimulus." In other words, pain and fear, or anxiety, from the patient's point of view, are inextricably enmeshed. To quote Beecher further, "It has been demonstrated experimentally that an increased fear of pain leads to overestimation of the intensity of painful stimuli." Dworkin (1970) demonstrated this point experimentally. He found

that pain as a stimulus, caused his subjects to respond with
greater anxiety and sensitivity to the stimulus in the
dental setting than in the laboratory. Grainger (1972) describes each dental appointment or procedure as a "crisis
situation for the patients."

Robinson (N.D.), studying pain as a motivating factor
in seeking care, differentiated between persons who were
pain-oriented and those who were not. Pain-oriented persons
were defined as those seeking care only to obtain relief of
pain. He found that 70% of the pain-oriented group admitted
waiting until they experienced pain before going for care
and 83% were actually experiencing pain at the time of his
survey.

White (1970) describes the public as being "absolutely
terrified" of dental visits. He states that because of
these fears, an estimated "10 to 12 million Americans studi-
ously avoid any sort of professional dental care."

The Division of Dentistry's national surveys of 1959,
1968, and 1972 asked three questions having to do with the
frequencies and reasons for dental visits pertinent to the
role of pain in preventive care. The 1959 survey demonstrated that 55% of the respondents reported going to the
dentist only when they needed to go and of these, 52% went
only when experiencing pain. Another 48% sought care when
they thought there might be a dental problem. Of the total
sample, (N=1,861) 43% said they visited the dentist for a
check-up.

The 1968 survey revealed that 20% of the sample (N=
1482) sought care only because their teeth ached or hurt,
or they thought there might be a problem, but 20% also reported attending for check-ups. The figures have scarcely
changed for the 1972 survey (N=1613). Twenty-two percent
visited the dentist because of toothache or possible other
trouble, and only 24% felt it was time for a check-up.

The 1968 survey also asked those who had made relatively infrequent visits to give their reasons for not making a
visit at least once a year. Five percent of these sometime
patients replied that they were afraid of dentists or did
not like dentists. The 1959 survey showed that 24% of the
respondents gave fear of pain as a reason for not seeing a

dentist when they believed they should have. Eight other
reasons were given also, but one might argue that being too
busy, believing the condition not serious, not wanting to
bother the dentist, inability to get an appointment at a
convenient time, not knowing a good dentist, or living too
far from the dentist, are mere rationalizations which allow
denial of the reason--fear of pain. That Kegeles (1963)
found a negative correlation between anxiety and fear of
pain and preventive dental visits emphasizes the need to
explore further, and particularly to explore among the vast
numbers who avoid all preventive dental and health care.

I could go on and cite many more studies which suggest
that the dental situation is feared and identified with pain.
Hence, the assumption by most health professionals that the
public is generally fearful, though not always acting in
terms of their fear, appears to be justified. Yet this
assumption has not been documented epidemiologically. The
self-reporting of survey respondents seem to be our only
source of information at this time. And we all know about
the problems of validity when self-reports require revealing
information about the self which the individual would rather
not admit or even consider. Projective test findings correlated with frequency of dental visits or dental status
might provide an index more reflective of the extent of
fear of dental pain.

Despite what we do know about pain and fear of pain,
we do not know enough about the extent to which the public
is governed by fear of pain, nor do we know all the ramifications of the barriers imposed by fear of pain on preventive dental or other health behaviors. We do not know
enough about how it affects the public health. Most study
has been concerned with perception of pain or reaction to
pain of individuals who are submitting to professional care.
The fearful patient, who comes for preventive treatment
even though reluctantly, does come and is not really a public health problem.

The problem of fear of pain is compounded because pain
can both motivate and inhibit. Whether it does one or the
other may depend on a particular configuration of variables,
i.e., the particular interactions of psychological, social,
and cultural factors. We have evidence that fear of pain
motivates for prevention when the individual believes he is

likely to have more pain through neglect than he is through regular examination. This interpretation is suggested by the "health belief model" of Hochbaum (1959), Haefner, Rosenstock, Kegeles, Kirscht (1966) and their associates, which deals with beliefs of susceptibility, seriousness of disease, and confidence in the benefits of regular care. Tash et al. (1969) tested a series of hypotheses suggested by this model, among them, the hypothesis that persons who believed that dental care would cause pain would be less likely to seek preventive dental care than persons who did not so believe. Though the data were interpreted as tending to support the hypothesis, only a 7% difference in reported preventive behavior existed between those fearing pain and those not fearing it. So the question remains, when does pain motivate and when does it inhibit? We have too little knowledge of the inhibiting configurations. We need also to identify the crucial variables that play a part in establishing pain and fear of pain as inhibitors of preventive health behaviors.

Actually, we need to ask a series of questions about motivation versus inhibition. e.g., at what age is pain, as a motivator or inhibitor to preventive care, most likely to be established? What factors, either cultural, social, or psychological are most likely to contribute to the establishment of motivation or inhibition? Which groups within the population are most likely to become either motivated or inhibited?

Some investigators have been most concerned with the psychological processes involved in the establishment of fear of pain. For example, Mackenzie, in a 1968 review of the literature on the psychodynamics of pain, stated that the patient's perception of pain "is more influential in determining his subsequent actions than the noxious stimulus itself." His review identified five classes of variables which he believes affect the perception of pain. These are: cultural variables; personal history variables; personality variables; emotional, and cognitive variables. I shall deal with the cultural variables later in this paper. As far as present data is concerned personal history variables seem to be most relevant to the perceptual, emotional, and cognitive elements which are all involved in learning experiences. Moreover, the evidence is that the learning related to perception of pain influences the ability to tolerate

pain. Tolerance to pain is obviously a factor influencing
the motivation or inhibition to seek preventive care and is
one that has also been shown to be psychologically, socio-
logically, and culturally dependent. According to Beecher
(1959), Petrovich (1958), and many others, early experience
with pain sets the level of tolerance for future pain experiences. Early traumatic episodes with the dentist or other
health personnel without compensating reward may lower tolerance and increase inhibition--or, again depending upon
other factors operating during the early experience, may
raise the level of tolerance and decrease inhibition. Not
only is a tolerance level to pain established, but a perceptual consciousness is created which may or may not be a
barrier to preventive action (Grainger, 1972). When in-
tolerance or a low tolerance to pain is clearly the case,
how to deal with the problem may be obvious. For example,
raising the tolerance level and changing the perceptual
consciousness should diminish the role of pain as an inhibitor. A number of techniques have been developed to
raise the tolerance level of pain. Among these are methods
to divert the patient's attention from pain (Kanfer and
Goldfoot, 1966), methods to prepare the patient for what to
expect (Egbert, et al., 1964), hypnotism (Barber, 1963),
audio-analgesia (Gardner, et al., 1960), desensitization
(Lang, 1966), behavior modeling (Rosenberg, 1974; Adelson,
et al., 1972), and a variety of other anxiety reducing
procedures (Weisenberg and Epstein, 1973).

Since early personal experiences may be critical in
establishing a set toward dental or medical care, the best
solution to the problem may be to direct our efforts toward
children in preventing or controlling the initial fear of
pain. Colchamira's (1970) exploratory investigation of
children's concepts and fear of dental care showed that
"fear of the dentist did not increase significantly after
the first dental visit," but there was a trend for increasing "pre-first-dental-visit fear" as a child got older. In
this study, projective test results suggest that an inner,
underlying, nonspecific fear of pain might provide inhibition later in life to seeking medical or dental care. The
first dental visit, itself, seemed not to be fear-producing,
rather the converse. If a child's first visit occurred at
a very early age, fear of dental care seemed not to develop.
The author attributes this to the enlightening effect on
the children's attitudes of knowledge through a rewarding

personal experience. Unfortunately, it has not always been
possible to expose pre-school children of all segments of
the population to the dentist early enough to avoid an
unpleasant first encounter and the development of fear of
dental pain. (Perhaps under Medicaid and possibly a future
National Health Insurance Plan, the removal of economic
barriers will lead to improvement in this condition, with
salutory results.)

These findings, together with others, suggest that the
dental situation itself, provides the most important initial, motivating or inhibiting contribution to fear of pain.
Anxiety induced stress about what to expect may cause a
small amount of pain to be experienced as severe (Beecher,
1959). Early frequent, and routine visits to the dentist
tend to dispel the anxiety produced by "fear of the unknown."
In New Zealand, the school dental nurse's procedures are
routinized to the extent of seeming compulsive, and thus
the children undergoing these procedures are never surprised.
They know exactly what to expect. One might postulate that
because of the influence on dental values of the dental care
system for children in New Zealand, the children are willing
to accept some pain.

The influential role of socioeconomic status in determining preventive dental utilization and other types of
preventive health measures, is by now generally accepted.
Cost of care, fairly regularly turns up as a partial cause
for under-utilization of preventive services among the
lower socioeconomic groups. But more than the cost of care
interferes with the seeking of regular preventive care.
That other inhibitors may be operating on the social class
level is indicated by the results of Nikias' (1968) study
of utilization and prepaid dental services. Even when
economic factors were reduced through prepaid dental services, large differences occurred in the frequency of dental
visits according to social class. Preventive care was available without the economic burden, but the lower socioecon-
mic groups did not change their patterns of utilization.
It's possible that one or more inhibiting variables were
collaboratively influencing behavior. e.g., Rayner (1969)
found that lower SES children experienced their first dental
visit as long as two to three or more years later than upper
SES children. Visits were more likely to have been precipi-
tated by acute need, i.e. toothache--perhaps requiring

extraction. The first dental encounter, then, was probably painful, thereby fixing an expectation of pain for all dental visits thereafter.

Sub-conditions of lower socioeconomic status contribute to the defining of dental care as painful, e.g., lower level of education. The 1959 survey showed that a significantly greater number of individuals educated below the college level, admitted not seeing a dentist because they feared the treatment might be painful. Moreover, 76% of those having only a grammar school education had never heard of the high-speed, painless dental drill; 48% of those with high school had never heard, but only 24% with a college education were unaware of the advances against pain in dentistry.

Perhaps the cultural variables responsible for the inhibition to seeking preventive care are most challenging. Challenging, first because we are not sure of what the inhibiting attributes might consist, and second because to change these may require profound modifications of perceptions, beliefs and values of large groups in the population. Or, more realistically, may require profound changes in how health professionals deal with these groups. Cultural values are obviously a factor. Definition of pain, the threat of pain and what it means, have been shown to be related to culturally dependent values. Nowhere is this seen more clearly than in the studies of Zborowski (1969) or Zola (1966) cited earlier in this paper.

Among the cultural variables, Zborowski's culturally determined attitudes of "pain acceptance" and "pain expectancy" seem pertinent to a concept of inhibitory reaction. Perceptual variation is most certainly embedded in the value system of a culture. The place of health in the culture's hierarchy of values certainly affects preventive health behavior. If health is not high in this scale of values, fear of pain is more likely to inhibit. If health is valued, then fear of pain, its meaning and consequences motivate--this last is a corollary of the "health beliefs model" mentioned earlier. Where the acceptance of pain is also a value, the fear and anxiety so often associated with pain may be minimized. This could be in the interest of preventive dental or medical care in that the fear or anxiety element does not exert an inhibitory influence.

Expectation of pain per se and <u>acceptance of pain as a value</u> differ. The former carries with it the connotation that one also will accept the pain. Only the future oriented time dimension seems to separate the two. Again, if health is valued, then the expectation of pain does not inhibit seeking preventive care. It should be emphasized, however, that health must really be valued, not merely lip-service be paid to the concept. Continuing and future health must be visualized as rewards for overcoming fear and accepting some pain.

But these last few statements are mainly common sense hypotheses. Zborowski's (1969), Antonovsky's (1970), and Zola's (1966) work on ethnic groups, though related, are not directed toward confirmation of these hypotheses. There is no existing research directed toward scientific support for them.

I admit to having dealt too briefly with the foregoing, and not at all with other aspects of pain as it relates to preventive health behavior. I have not dealt with the psychoanalytic approach to the problem--largely because psychoanalysis seems not to be practical for dealing with masses of people who seldom or never get to the dentist. The psychoanalytic approach emphasizes the dentist-patient relationship and may be useful for helping individuals already in dental therapy, and it may be useful in encouraging continuing preventive care. On the other hand, the highly specialized training needed to use psychoanalytic techniques effectively may limit its use in the dental situation.

Nor have I discussed the role of fear of pain in terms of intermediate and older age groups. There is some information from the 1959 survey which was mentioned earlier and some from an ongoing retirement history study (Irelan, 1972) being carried out by the Office of Research and Statistics of the Social Security Administration of HEW. Apart from these two sources, data is very meager. The survey data suggests that very little difference exists between the ages of 20 and 64 years in the percentage of persons who admit avoiding care. Approximately one out of four avoid care because of fear of pain. Of persons 65 and older, only 18% admitted fear of pain as a reason for not seeking care. Of course, lack of dentition in the older group may account for the 7% drop in admissions of fear.

The retirement study sample consisting of 11,153 persons, both married and single men and single women, aged 58-63, provides information on the postponement of needed dental and medical care. Approximately 30% of the total sample deferred dental care. Moreover, this figure is larger than that of any other health category. Approximately 15% gave fear as a reason for postponing care.

And finally, I would like to summarize by reiterating the point which I hope I have made throughout this paper-- that is, that we do not know _enough_ about the role of pain as a deterrent to preventive health practices and care. We do not have enough information on fear of pain as an inhibitor. We accept the assumption that pain is a deterrent to care but we have the most understanding of it as a motivator. Yet, to best serve the public, we should understand the dynamics of pain and the social and _cultural_ effects of pain as an inhibitor. We need more accurate statistics on the number of persons who avoid preventive care, more objective means for determining the depth, significance, and reality of pain as a deterrent to preventive care. And lastly, we need to search for the best methods for reaching those members of the population who escape the web of health educational and care systems because they fear pain.

REFERENCES

Adelson, R., Liebert, R.M., Poulos, R.W. and Herskovitz, A. A modeling film to reduce children's fear of dental treatment. Paper read before the Behavioral Science Section, International Association of Dental Research, Las Vegas, Nevada, March 24, 1972. Abstract #266.

Antonovsky, A. and Katz, R. The model dental patient - an empirical study of preventive health behavior. _Social Science and Medicine_, 1970, 4, 367-380.

Barber, T.X. The effects of 'hypnosis' on pain: a critical review of experimental and clinical findings. _Psychosomatic Medicine_, 1963, 25, 303-333.

Beecher, H.K. Quantifiable expressions of anxiety. _Measurement of Subjective Responses_, Chapter 15, 1959, 342-351.

Colchamiro, S. The development of the child's concepts and fear of dental care. Submitted as the fulfillment of the requirements of graduation "with honors" at Harvard School of Dental Medicine (May, 1970). Presented at the 110th Annual Session of the American Dental Association, 1969.

Cole, L. Attitudes toward dental treatment: a motivational analysis. The Journal of the Philippine Dental Association, 1961, 14, 20-24.

Dworkin, S.F. Pain responsivity and its relationship to situational context and body-concept. Dissertation Abstracts International, 1970, 31, 1533-B.

Egbert, L.D., Battit, G.E., Welsh, E.E. and Bartlet, M.K. Reduction of post-operative pain by encouragement and instruction to patients: a study of doctor-patient rapport. New England Journal of Medicine, 1964, 270, 825-827.

Freeman, H.E. and Lambert, Jr., C. Preventive dental behavior of urban mothers. Journal of Health and Human Behavior, 1965, 6, 141-147.

Gardner, W.J., Licklider, J.C.R. and Weiss, A.F. Suppression of pain by sound. Science, 1960, 132, 32-33.

Green, L.W. Status identity and preventive health behavior. Pacific Health Education Reports, University of California, Berkeley and University of Hawaii, Honolulu, 1970, 1.

Gochman, D.S. Some correlates of children's health beliefs and potential health behavior. Journal of Health & Social Behavior, 1971, 12, 148-154.

Grainger, J.K. Perception: its meaning, significance and control in dental procedures Part II. psychological aspects. Australian Dental Journal, 1972, 17, 110-116.

Hetherington, R.W. and Hopkins, C.E. Symptom sensitivity: its social and cultural correlates. Health Services Research, 1969, 4, 63-75.

Hochbaum, G.M. Some principles of health behavior. Proceedings of the 1959 Biennial Conference of the State and Territorial Dental Directors with the Public Health Service and the Children's Bureau, April 21-23, Washington, D.C. U. S. Department of Health, Education, and Welfare, PHS Publication No. 698, p. 17. Washington, D.C.: Government Printing Office, 1959.

Kanfer, F.H. and Goldfoot, D.A. Self-control and tolerance of noxious stimulation. Psychological Reports, 1966, 18, 79.

Kegeles, S.S. Some motives for seeking preventive dental care. Journal of the American Dental Association, 1963, 67, 90-98.

Kirscht, J.P., Haefner, D.P., Kegeles, S.S. and Rosenstock, I.M. A national study of health beliefs. Journal of Health and Human Behavior, 1966, 7, 248-254.

Lambert, C. and Freeman, H.E. The clinic habit. New Haven,
    Connecticut: College and University Press, 1967.
Lang, P.J. Experimental studies of fear reduction. Journal
    of Dental Abstracts, 1966, 45, 1618.
Mackenzie, R.S. Psychodynamics of pain. Journal of Oral
    Medicine, 1968, 23, 75-84.
Mechanic, D. The influence of mothers on their children's
    health attitudes and behavior. Pediatrics, 1964, 33,
    444-453.
Newman, J.J. and Anderson, O.W. Patterns of Dental Service
    Utilization in the United States: A Nationwide Social
    Survey. Center for Health Administration Studies, Uni-
    versity of Chicago, Research Series 30, 1972.
Nikias, M.K. Social class and the use of dental care under
    prepayment. Medical Care, 1968, 6, 381-393.
O'Shea, R.M. and Gray, S.B. Dental patients' attitudes and
    behavior concerning prevention. Public Health Reports,
    1968, 83, 405-410.
Petrovich, D.V. The pain apperception test: psychological
    correlates of pain perception. Journal of Clinical Psy-
    chology, 1958, 14, 367-374.
Pettibone, T.J. and Solis, Jr., E. Dental health care models
    of southwest cultures. Education Research Center, New
    Mexico State University, 1973.
Richardson, J.T. Fear: a psychological and a dental prob-
    lem. South Carolina Dental Journal, 1972, 30, 27-31.
Robinson, E. Pain as a motivating factor in seeking dental
    care. Department of Community Dentistry, University of
    Michigan (N.D.).
Rosenberg, H.M. Behavior modification for the child dental
    patient. Journal of Dentistry for Children, 1974, 41,
    31-34.
Rosenstock, I.M. Why people use health services. The Mil-
    bank Memorial Fund Quarterly, 1966, 44, 94-127.
Tash, R.H., O'Shea, R.M., and Cohen, L.K. Testing a pre-
    ventive-symptomatic theory of dental health behavior.
    American Journal of Public Health, 1969, 59, 514-521.
Weisenberg, M. Behavioral motivation. Journal of Perio-
    dontology, 1973, 44, 489-499.
Weisenberg, M. and Epstein, D. Patient training as an al-
    ternative to general anesthesia. New York State Dental
    Journal, 1973, 39, 610-613.

White, W.L. Public beliefs and attitudes concerning pre-
    ventive dentistry. Paper read before the 14th Annual
    Meeting on Dental Health Workshop. Title: Motivation
    in Preventive Dentistry. Sponsored by the Missouri
    Dental Association, January 18-19, 1970.
Zborowski, M. People in Pain. San Franscico, California:
    Jossey-Bass Inc., Publishers, 1969.
Zola, I. K. Culture and symptoms--an analysis of patients'
    presenting complaints. American Sociological Review,
    1966, 31, 615-630.

BIBLIOGRAPHY

Adelson, R., Liebert, R.M., Poulos, R.W. and Herskovitz, A.
    A modeling film to reduce children's fear of dental
    treatment. Paper read before the Behavioral Science
    Section, International Association of Dental Research,
    Las Vegas, Nevada, March 24, 1972. Abstract #266.
Agle, D.P., Baum, G.L., Chester, E.H. and Wendt, M. Multi-
    discipline treatment of chronic pulmonary insufficiency
    1. Psychologic aspects of rehabilitation. Psychosomatic
    Medicine, 1973, 35, 41-49.
Antonovsky, A. and Kats, R. The model dental patient - an
    empirical study of preventive health behavior. Social
    Science and Medicine, 1970, 4, 367-380.
Antonovsky, A. A model to explain visits to the doctor:
    with specific reference to the case of Israel. Journal
    of Health & Social Behavior, 1972, 13, 446-454.
Bailey, P.M., Talbot, A. and Taylor, P. A comparison of
    maternal anxiety levels with anxiety levels manifested
    in the child dental patient. Journal of Dentistry for
    Children, 1973, 40, 25-32.
Barber, T.X. The effects of "Hypnosis" on pain: a critical
    review of experimental and clinical findings. Psycho-
    somatic Medicine, 1963, 25, 303-333.

Becker, M.H., Drachman, R.H. and Kirscht, P. A new approach
    to explaining sick-role behavior in low-income popula-
    tions. American Journal of Public Health, 1974, 64, 205-
    216.
Beecher, H.K. Quantifiable expressions of anxiety. Measure-
    ment of Subjective Responses. New York: Oxford Univer-
    sity Press, 1959, Chapter 15, 342-351.
Brown, R.A. and Fader, K. The generality of pain sensiti-
    vity and its relationship to personality. Tufts Univer-
    sity, Department of Social Dentistry, Buffalo Project,
    September 1, 1971.
Bulman, J.S., Slack, G.L., Richards, N.D. & Willcocks, A.J.
    A survey of the dental health and attitudes towards
    dentistry in two communities - Part 2.--dental data.
    British Dental Journal, 1968, 124, 549-554.
Bulman, J.S., Slack, L., Richards, N.D. & Willcocks, A.J.
    A survey of the dental health and attitudes towards
    dentistry in two communities - Part 3.--comparison of
    dental and sociological data. British Dental Journal,
    1968, 125, 102-106.
Colchamiro, S. The development of the child's concepts and
    fear of dental care. Submitted as the fulfillment of the
    requirements of graduation "with honors" at Harvard
    School of Dental Medicine - 5/70. Presented as part of
    the: 110th Annual Session of the ADA 10/1969 - Annual
    Meeting of the IADR 3/70 and Annual Meeting of the Mass.
    Dental Society 5/70.
Cole, L. Attitudes toward dental treatment: a motivational
    analysis. The Journal of the Philippine Dental Associa-
    tion, 1961, 14, 20-24.
Current estimates - from the Health Interview Survey -
    United States - 1972. Vital and Health Statistics,
    Series 10, No. 85, page 25. U.S. Department of Health,
    Education, and Welfare, Public Health Serivce, Health
    Resources Administration, National Center for Health
    Statistics, Rockville, Md. 1973.
DeFee, J.F. and Himlestein, P. Children's fear in a dental
    situation as a function of birth order. The Journal of
    Genetic Psychology, 1969, 115, 253-255.
Dental visits - volume and interval since last visit -
    United States - 1969. Vital and Health Statistics,
    Series 10, No. 76, pages 1 and 5. U.S. Department of
    Health, Education, and Welfare, Public Health Service,
    Health Services and Mental Health Administration, National
    Center for Health Statistics, Rockville, Md. 1972.

DiBona, C. The relationship between fear and intelligence in the child patient. The New York Journal of Dentistry. 1973, 43, 52-56.

Dickson, S. Class attitudes to dental treatment. The British Journal of Sociology, 1968, 19, 206-211.

Dworkin, S.F. Pain responsivity and its relationship to situational context and body-concept. Dissertation Abstracts International, 1970, 31, #3, 1533-B.

Egbert, L.D., Battit, G.E. Welsh, E.E. and Bartlet, M.K. Reduction of post-operative pain by encouragement and instruction to patients: a study of doctor-patient rapport. New England Journal of Medicine, 1964, 270, 825-827.

Ellenbogen, B.L., Lowe, G.D. and Danley, R.A. The diffusion of two preventive health practices. Inquiry, 1968, 5, 62-71.

Forsberg, A. Tandvardsskrack [Fear of Dental Treatment]. Svensk Tandlakare-Tidskrift, 1966, 59, 147-159.

Frazier, P., Jenny, J. and Bagramian, R.A. Parents' descriptions of barriers faced and strategies used to obtain dental care. Journal of Public Health Dentistry. 1974, 34, 22-38.

Freeman, H.E. and Lambert, C.,Jr. Preventive dental behavior of urban mothers. Journal of Health and Human Behavior. 1965, 6, 141-147.

Gale, E.N. Fears of the dental situation. Journal of Dental Research, 1972, 51, 964-966.

Gardner, W.J., Licklider, J.C.R. and Weiss, A.F. Suppression of pain by sound. Science, 1960, 132, 32-33.

Gochman, D.S. Some correlates of children's health beliefs and potential health behavior. Journal of Health and Social Behavior, 1971, 12, 148-154.

Gochman, D.S. Some steps towards a psychological matrix for health behavior. Canadian Journal of Behavioral Science/ Revue Canadienne Des Sciences Du Comportement, 1971, 3, 88-101.

Gonzales, L. and Silverstein, S.J. Make the dental clinic "a nice place to visit" (allaying patients' fears about a dental clinic, especially in a poverty community, will make dental care all the more effective). Dental Student, 1973, 51, 26-27.

Gordon, D.A., Terdal, L. and Sterling, E. The use of modeling and desensitization in the treatment of a phobic child patient. Journal of Dentistry for Children, 1974, 41, 22-25.

Grainger, J.K. Perception: its meaning, significance and control in dental procedures. Part II. psychological aspects. Australian Dental Journal, 1972, 17, 110-116.

Green, L.W. Status identity and preventive health beahvior. Pacific Health Education Reports, No. 1, University of California, Berkeley and University of Hawaii, Honolulu, 1970.

Haefner, D.P. and Kirscht, J.P. Motivational and behavioral effects of modifying health beliefs. Public Health Reports, 1970, 85, 478-484.

Hetherington, R.W. and Hopkins, C.E. Symptom sensitivity: its social and cultural correlates. Health Services Research, 1969, 4, 63-75.

Hochbaum, G.M. Some principles of health behavior. Proceedings of the 1959 Biennial Conference of the State and Territorial Dental Directors with the Public Health Service and the Children's Bureau, April 21-23, Washington, D.C. U. S. Department of Health, Education, and Welfare, PHS Publication No. 698, p. 17. Washington, D.C.: Government Printing Office, 1959.

Howitt, J.W. and Stricker, G. The influence of age, sex, intelligence and modified environment upon children's reaction to tooth pain. New York State Dental Journal, 1963, 29, 262-264.

Howitt, J.W. and Stricker, G. Physiological response measures of child dental patients. Paper read before the International Association of Dental Research, Toronto, Canada, 1965.

Janis, I.L. Effects of fear arousal on attitude change: recent developments in theory and experimental research. In L. Berkowitz (Ed.) Advances in Experimental Social Psychology. New York: Academic Press, 1967, 3, 166-222.

Janis, I.L. Psychological Stress. New York: John Wiley & Sons, Inc. 1958.

Kanfer, F.H. and Goldfoot, D.A. Self-control and tolerance of noxious stimulation. Psychological Reports, 1966, 18, 79-85.

Kaplan, R.I. Preventive dentistry--fact or fad? Journal of the American College of Dentists, 1973, 40, 217-224.

Kegeles, S.S. Some motives for seeking preventive dental care. Journal of the American Dental Association, 1963, 67, 90-98.

Kirscht, J.P., Haefner, D.P., Kegeles, S.S., and Rosenstock, I.M. A national study of health beliefs. University of Michigan, Ann Arbor, August 1961. (Mimeographed)

Kleinknecht, R.A., Klepac, R.K. and Alexander, L.D.   Origins
and characteristics of fear of dentistry.   Journal of the
American Dental Association, 1973, 86, 842-848.
Koenigsberg, R. and Johnson, R.   Child behavior during se-
quential dental visits.   Journal of the American Dental
Association, 1972, 85, 128-132.
Kutscher, A.H. and Kutscher, H.W.   Evaluation of the Hardy-
Wolff-Goodell pain threshold apparatus and technique:
review of the literature.   International Record of Medi-
cine, 1957, 70, 202-230.
Lamb, D.H. and Plant, R.   Patient anxiety in the dentist's
office.   Journal of Dental Research, 1972, 51, 986-989.
Lambert, C. and Freeman. H.E.   The Clinic Habit.   New Haven,
Connecticut: College and University Press, 1967.
Lang, P.J.   Experimental studies of fear reduction.   Journal
of Dental Abstracts, 1966, 45, 1618.
Lazarus, R.S.   Some principles of psychological stress and
their relation to dentistry.   Journal of Dental Abstracts,
1966, 45, 1620-1626.
Leventhal, H.   Fear appeals and persuasion: the differentia-
tion of a motivational construct.   American Journal of
Public Health, 1971, 61, 1208-1224.
Likeman, P.R.   A general review of the study of pain.   Edin-
burgh Dental Hospital Gazette, 1972, 12, 9-13.
Ludwig, E.G. and Gibson, G.   Self perception of sickness
and the seeking of medical care.   Journal of Health and
Social Behavior, 1969, 10, 125-133.
Mackenzie, R.S.   Psychodynamics of pain.   Journal of Oral
Medicine, 1968, 23, 75-84.
Mandel, I.D.   What is preventive dentistry?   Journal of
Preventive Dentistry, 1974, 1, 25-29.
Mechanic, D.   The influence of mothers on their children's
health attitudes and behavior.   Pediatrics, 1964, 33,
444-453.
Meichenbaum, D.H.   Examination of model characteristics in
reducing avoidance behavior.   Journal of Personality and
Social Psychology, 1971, 17, 298-307.
Miller, J. and Swallow, J.N.   Dental pain and health.   Pub-
lic Health (London), 1970, 85, 46-50.
Newman, J.J. and Anderson, O.W.   Patterns of dental service
utilization in the United States: a nationwide social
survey.   Center for Health Administration Studies, University of Chicago, Research Series 30, 1972.

Nikias, M.K.   Social class and the use of dental care under prepayment. Medical Care, 1968, 6, 381-393.

O'Shea, R.M. and Gray, S.B.   Dental patients' attitudes and behavior concerning prevention. Public Health Reports, 1968, 83, 405-410.

Oster, J.   Recurrent abdominal pain, headache and limb pains in children and adolescents. Pediatrics, 1972, 50, 429-436.

Petrovich, D.V.   The pain apperception test: psychological correlates of pain perception. Journal of Clinical Psychology, 1958, 14, 367-374.

Pettibone, T.J. and Solis, E., Jr.   Dental Health Care Models of Southwest Cultures.   Educational Research Center, New Mexico State University, December 1973.

Pizano, A.S.   Pain in Dentistry (Utilization of Libman's Test).   (translated from Spanish).

Plasschaert, A.J.M. and Konig, K.G.   The effect of information and motivation towards dental health, and of fluoride tablets on caries in school children.   I.   increment over the initial 2-year experimental period.   International Dental Journal, 1974, 24, 50-65.

Reeder, L.G. and Berkanovic, E.   Sociological concomitants of health orientations: a partial replication of Suchman.   Journal of Health & Social Behavior, 1973, 14, 134-143.

Richards, N.D., Willcocks, A.J., Bulman, J.S. and Slack, L. A survey of the dental health and attitudes towards dentistry in two communities.   British Dental Journal, 1965, 118, 199-205.

Richardson, T.   Fear: a psychological and a dental problem. South Carolina Dental Journal, 1972, 30, 27-31.

Robinson, E.   Pain as a motivating factor in seeking dental care.   Department of Community Dentistry, University of Michigan (N.D.)

Rogers, R.W. & Thistlethwaite, D.L.   Effects of fear arousal and reassurance on attitude change.   Journal of Personality and Social Psychology, 1970, 15, 227-233.

Rosenbaum, V.   Whatever happened to those teen-age dropouts? Dental Economics, 1974, 64, 35-39.

Rosenberg, M.   Behavioral modification for the child dental patient.   Journal of Dentistry for Children, 1974, 41, 31-34.

Rosenstock, I.M.   Why people use health services.   The Milbank Memorial Fund Quarterly, 1966, 44, 94-127.

Samuels, J.J. Behaviors and attitudes: implications for dental health education. Dental Hygiene, 1973, 47, 149-154.

Schanche, D.A. Dentistry's new approach to chasing pain. Virginia Dental Journal, 1973, 50, 7-14.

Shaw, C.T. Class characteristics of supporters and rejectors of basic health measures. Social Science and Medicine, 1970, 4, 411-415.

Shuval, J. A comparison of Israeli and American findings. Israel Study of Social and Psychological Factors in Dental Health. (Preliminary Draft).

Shuval, J.T. Preventive dental behavior in Israel: some contrasts between a profession population and its clients. Medical Care, 1971, 9, 345-351.

Steele, J.L. and McBroom, W.H. Conceptual and empirical dimensions of health behavior. Journal of Health and Social Behavior, 1972, 13, 382-392.

Stricker, G. Psychological issues pertaining to malocclusion. American Journal of Orthodontics, 1970, 58, 276-283.

Stricker, G. and Howitt, J.W. Physiological recording during simulated dental appointments. The New York State Dental Journal, 1965, 31, 204-206.

Suchman, E.A. Ethnic and social factors in medical care orientation. Milbank Memorial Fund Quarterly, 1969, 47, 69-77.

Suchman, E.A. Preventive health behavior: a model for research on community health campaigns. Journal of Health and Social Behavior, 1967, 197-209.

Sumnicht, R.W. Research in preventive dentistry. Journal of the American Dental Association, 1969, 79, 1193-1201.

Tash, R.H., O'Shea, R.M. and Cohen, L.K. Testing a preventive-symptomatic theory of dental health behavior. American Journal of Public Health, 1969, 59, 514-521.

Thomas, R. Attitudes towards dental treatment and dental surgeons. Probe, 1965, 16, 4-7.

Todes, C.J. The child and the dentist: a psychoanalytical view. British Journal of Medical Psychology, 1972, 45, 45-55.

Weisenberg, M. Behavioral motivation. Journal of Periodontology, 1973, 44, 489-499.

Weisenberg, M. and Epstein, D. Patient training as an alternative to general anesthesia. New York State Dental Journal, 1973, 39, 610-613.

Weisenberg, M., Kreindler, M.L. and Schachat, R. Relation-
    ship of the Dental Anxiety Scale to the State-Trait
    Anxiety Inventory. Journal of Dental Research, 1974, 53,
    946.
White, W.L. Public beliefs and attitudes concerning pre-
    ventive dentistry. Paper read before the 14th Annual
    Workshop on Dental Health. Workshop Title: Motivation
    in Preventive Dentistry. Sponsored by the Missouri
    Dental Association, January 18-19, 1970.
White, Jr., W.C., Akers, J., Green, J. and Yates, D. Use
    of imitation in the treatment of dental phobia in early
    childhood. A preliminary report. Journal of Dentistry
    for Children, 1974, 41, 26-30.
Who's afraid? Not children who 'play dentist'. The Journal
    of Dental Practice, 1972, 48, 37.
Wilkins, W. Desensitization: social and cognitive factors
    underlying the effectiveness of Wolpe's procedure.
    Psychological Bulletin, 1971, 76, 311-315.
Woodrow, K.M., Friedman, G.D., Siegelaub, A.B. and Collen,
    M.F. Pain tolerance: differences according to age, sex
    and race. Psychosomatic Medicine, 1972, 34, 548-556.
Wright, G.Z. and Alpern, G.D. Variables influencing chil-
    dren's cooperative behavior at the first dental visit.
    ASDC Journal of Dentistry for Children, 1971, 37, 124-
    128.
Wright, G.Z., Alpern, G.D. and Leake, J.L. A cross-valida-
    tion of variables affecting children's cooperative be-
    haviour. Journal of the Canadian Dental Association,
    1973, 39, 268-273.
Wright, G.Z., Alpern, G.D. and Leake, J.L. The modifiability
    of maternal anxiety as it relates to children's coopera-
    tive dental behavior. ASDC Journal of Dentistry for
    Children, 1973, 39, 265-271.
Zborowski, M. People in Pain. San Francisco, Calif.:
    Jossey-Bass Inc., Publishers, 1969.
Zola, I.K. Culture and symptoms--an analysis of patients'
    presenting complaints. American Sociological Review,
    1966, 31, 615-630.

TEACHING BEHAVIORAL PAIN CONTROL TO HEALTH PROFESSIONALS

Matisyohu Weisenberg

University of Connecticut Health Center

Farmington, Connecticut

The goal of this presentation is to describe an approach to teaching a comprehensive view of pain control that was developed over the past four years. The course "The Perception and Control of Pain" was taught as a four week elective during preclinical training to a combined group of medical and dental students. It represented for most students the only opportunity for formal instruction in a broad view of pain that included a behavioral perspective and behavioral techniques of control. It was both didactic and experiential to the extent allowable.

COURSE OBJECTIVES

The formal course objectives were:

1. To achieve an understanding of the complexity of the pain reaction.
2. To review the social, psychological, pharmacological and physiological dimensions involved in the reaction to pain.
3. To acquire knowledge of psychological and other techniques for the reduction of pain perception.

The basic underlying philosophy of the course is that pain perception and reactions are complex phenomena for which many questions still remain to be answered. No single discipline has all the answers. Treatment, too, includes many approaches. No one single approach is best for all patients under all circumstances.

113

COURSE ORGANIZATION

The course includes a review of physiological mechanisms as well as pharmacological and surgical approaches to
pain control. However, the major emphasis is on social and
psychological factors that affect the perception and reaction to pain. Consistent with a multidisciplinary orientation experts are brought in to teach their areas of specialization. This past year's faculty included two psychologists, a neurophysiologist, a pharmacologist, a neurosurgeon
and an anesthesiologist. In previous years guest lecturers
from outside the university were also included, e.g., James
Hardy who lectured on his basic pain research.

Class time is divided into a two hour seminar and a
one hour laboratory session. The seminar is used for discussion of the didactic material. Lecturing is kept at a
minimum. The laboratory is used for teaching hypnosis,
deep-muscle relaxation techniques and the use of biofeedback procedures. The emphasis in the laboratory sessions
is to have students actually perform the procedures on one
another.

Outside the classroom students spend time in a variety
of clinical settings observing and later discussing in
class current pain control practices - both the good and
the bad. On the positive side students have the opportunity to learn from experienced providers how to introduce
patients to treatment, deal with their fears and use a
variety of pain control measures. On the negative side
students observe providers who act to suit their conve-
nience rather than to benefit their patients e.g., routine
use of general anesthesia instead of awake childbirth to
allow the obstetrician to go home. In some clinics the
only approach to pain control is medication. Patients are
told that if 10 aspirin do not relieve the pain, take 12.
No other approach is ever tried.

COURSE CONTENT (see appendix for sample course outline)

The course begins with a review of the physiological
mechanisms of pain. All students have already completed a
course on the central nervous system. They are thus familiar with basic neuroanatomy and physiology. The review
includes a discussion of theories of pain with an emphasis

on gate-control theory (Melzack and Wall, 1970). Although
there is disagreement regarding the correctness of the
wiring diagram of the gate-control theory, it still is the
most comprehensive and influential current theory of pain.
It is able to tie together many of the puzzling phenomena
of pain perception and control and best accounts for the
effects of psychological variables. It also leads to a
variety of techniques of control that have validity.

Defining pain can be very difficult. Sensory psychologists and physiologists have mostly viewed pain as a
separate sensation along with temperature and other cutaneous senses (Geldard, 1972; Kenshalo, 1971; Mountcastle,
1974; Hardy, Wolff and Goodell, 1952). Each author men-
tions that emotional factors are very important in affecting the reaction to pain. However, they then proceed to
an almost purely sensory discussion of pain. Sternbach
(1968) has defined pain as "...1) a personal, private sensation of hurt; 2) a harmful stimulus which signals impending tissue damage; 3) a pattern of responses which operates
to protect the organism from harm" (page 12).

Definitions of pain in stimulus-response terms are
inadequate clinically. There are examples of pain for
which no apparent stimuli can be demonstrated. Psychiatric
illness, especially depression, has been associated with
complaints of pain (Spear, 1967). Melzack (1973) has discussed examples such as causalgia or phantom limb where the
pain persists months after the tissue damage has healed.
Peripheral stimulus input does not adequately account for
central pain, while in chronic pain, the warning signal
notion does not seem appropriate.

Given all the limitations in defining pain, the course
follows Melzack and Wall (1970) in viewing pain as a psychological experience that includes a sensory component as
well as motivational-cognitive-affective components. Dwell-
ing on definitions is not just an intellectual exercise.
Its purpose is to avoid simplistic views of pain that
suggest simplistic treatment strategies often with disappointing outcomes. For example, viewing pain as any other
sensation suggests that there are straight forward pain
pathways. Surgical results, however, indicate a rather
disappointing record of success (c.f., Schurmann, 1972).

Viewing pain as a complex phenomena suggests a diversity

of strategies. Treatment may consist of reducing the aversive affective component of pain while leaving the sensory
component relatively intact. This can be achieved by use
of medication or by use of the principles of learning (c.f.,
Fordyce, Fowler, Lehman, and Delateur, 1968).

Despite the clinical limitations of the sensory psychologists and physiologists, they have made major contribu-
tions to the scientific analysis of pain. These contri-
butions are also discussed in the course. They include a
description of the qualities of pain (pricking, burning,
aching), the mapping of body sensitivity and the development of finely controlled methods of stimulation and
measurement that can be used in some clinical situations.

Pain measurement is at once one of the most difficult
as well as important tasks. It affects our ability to
understand the basic concepts of pain, to produce a proper
clinical diagnosis and to determine the effectiveness of
medication or other means of intervention. Time is spent
on discussion of the criteria for evaluating pain stimuli
for laboratory and clinical purposes. Distinctions are
made between threshold and tolerance and how these are
measured by different procedures in a variety of settings.

Once definitions of pain and methods of measurement
have been discussed, it becomes possible to examine the
social and psychological correlates of pain perception
and attempts at the experimental manipulation of pain.

Several points are kept in mind when evaluating the
results of these studies. Do these studies refer to pain
threshold or (the point where the sensation of pain is
first perceived) to pain tolerance (the point where the
person no longer wishes to receive any more stimulation or
go any higher)? Most studies, for example, do not find sex
differences for threshold but they do for tolerance. What
kind of pain stimulation is being used? Variations in these
studies include cutaneous pain from electric shock, the
relatively slow arising pain of cold water, the even slower
and more intense pain of muscle ischemia, and mechanical
pressure to produce deep pain.

That differences between different types of stimulation exist, is known. What is not always clear from the
literature is the nature of these differences. Beecher's

(1966) preference is for something that is affected by morphine. He therefore, chooses ischemic pain in his studies.
Hilgard (1973) found that hypnosis was differentially effective in changing physiological reactions for ischemic as
compared to cold water pain. What do these differences
mean? Such problems can make it difficult to draw clinically relevant conclusions from data dealing with correlates of pain perception and once more emphasize the complexity of pain reactions.

Studies of the experimental manipulation of pain seek
to define cause and effect relationships rather than simply
rely on correlational evidence. In the laboratory setting
it has been demonstrated how choice (Zimbardo, Cohen, Weisenberg, Dworkin and Firestone, 1966) and subject control (Staub,
Tursky and Schwartz, 1971) can increase pain tolerance.

Modeling is a short-hand vicarious means of teaching a
person the consequences of a behavior without necessitating
trial and error experience (Bandura, 1969). It has been
shown to have a pronounced effect on increasing pain tolerance as demonstrated in the laboratory (Craig and Weiss,
1971, Neufeld and Davidson, 1971). Distraction and attention processes also can have a profound effect on pain reactions. They can easily be manipulated by instructions
(c.f., Blitz and Dinnerstein, 1971).

Other approaches that have been shown to reduce pain
and stress include relaxation (Jacobson, 1938), hypnosis
(Hartland, 1971), desensitization, (Wolpe, 1973) and biofeedback (Miller, Barber, DiCara, Kamiya, et al, 1974). Each
laboratory approach has clinical implications to increase
pain tolerance. These are discussed during the seminar.

In the clinic, for example, too often there is a fear
of allowing patients some degree of control over the situation. Linn (1967) observed 27 dentists, their assistants
and 114 patients at two dental clinics to determine behaviors necessary in the doctor-patient relationship in order
for it to continue. The most important role for the patient
was conformity while that for the dentist was authority to
direct. Patients rarely directed or requested anything
from the dentist. Yet, allowing the patient some degree of
choice and control could probably have enhanced the reduction of patient distress and his ability to tolerate pain.

Preparation for aversive stimulation has been effectively used in the laboratory to reduce the distress of pain
stimulation. Neufeld and Davidson (1971) suggest that prior
rehearsal should be repeated over time prior to the aversive
event e.g., several sessions separated by a week's time.

Johnson (1973) and Johnson and Leventhal (1974) present laboratory and clinical evidence concerning the effectiveness of different types of preparations. Information
regarding the sensations to be experienced is more effective in reducing stress than only information regarding the
procedures to be used. Reducing the incogruency between
expectations and experience is one way of reducing anxiety
based on the fear of the unknown.

In their study of patients undergoing gastrointestinal
endoscopic examination it was found that the combination of
description of sensations and recommendations of coping behavior reduced the emotional reaction as measured by heart
rate and produced marked reduction in gagging.

Preparation for surgery has been credited with reducing severity of postoperative outcomes (Egbert, Battit,
Welch and Bartlett, 1964). What are the crucial ingredi-
ents that go into patient preparation? Janis (1958) has
emphasized anxiety.

Unfortunately, subsequent studies have not supported
Janis's emphasis on fear and anxiety, Cohen and Lazarus
(1973) have emphasized the importance of coping strategies
in dealing with the stress of surgery. Unlike Janis, they
feel that denial would be beneficial strategy to use when
the outcome is expected to be positive. Exactly which
mechanisms are involved may still be open to debate. It
seems that it may be some combination of anxiety reduction
and coping strategy through adequate preparation.

Beecher (1972) has argued that anxiety reduction not
only can make pain more tolerable but it is the major mode
of action of drugs that alleviate pain. Clinically, this
would mean that a combination of anxiety reduction and
coping strategies would increase the effectiveness of pain
medication. Thompson (1974), from the clinician's view,
has emphasized how important this preparation can be.
"Occasionally the dentist will learn that he can make some

patients more comfortable by the things he says and does
than by the medication he uses" (page 59).

Learning to cope with pain is important not only for
acute but for chronic pain as well. Chronic pain is a
more difficult problem for the clinician. Many of the out-
ward signs of acute pain are lacking and as Hackett (1967)
points out the physician often is at a loss to deal with
the pain and as a result ends up questioning the sanity of
his patient. The inability to deal with chronic pain also
encourages patients to seek relief elsewhere; often from
quacks who at least provide a sympathetic ear while relieving the patient of his money. These quacks can teach practitioners that there is more to medicine than surgery or
simply prescribing another pill (Gordon, 1966). Even though
there is no cure for many types of pain problems, it is
still possible to let the patient realize that he can be
taught how to deal with what he has. Everything will be
done to help him obtain as much as he can from life even
with his pain problem.

Spear (1967) has shown that pain is a common complaint
in psychiatric patients. Treating the underlying symptoms
seems to relieve the pain. Depression is very strongly
related to pain and anti-depressants can provide relief.
It should be pointed out, however, that so called psychogenic pain patients do not yield easily discernible patterns
in mental health tests. As Sternbach (1974) has shown,
both organic and psychogenic chronic pain sufferers yield
similar MMPI profiles. It, therefore, behooves health
providers to be a little more cautious in their quick pro-
nouncements and treatments. In any case whether the pain
is due to organic or psychogenic causes, for the patient it
is just as real. For the provider the difference would
come in his readiness to perform surgery or other drastic
procedures that might not help anyway.

Discussion of cultural differences emphasizes the
variety of reactions given by different groups of people
when in pain (c.f., Weisenberg, 1976). There is no one
"correct" way of reacting when in pain. Health providers
must therefore, not let preconceived notions of what is an
appropriate pain reaction prejudice their treatment (c.f.,
Pilowsky and Bond, 1969). Understanding cultural differences therefore can be useful in diagnosis and in deciding
a treatment strategy.

During the course, a few selected specific types of
pain problems are also discussed. Headache represents one
of the most common types of pain complaints (c.f., Dalessio,
1972). Several types of headaches also have strong behavioral components. Treatment strategy should deal with
these. Tension and migraine headache pain, for example,
been successfully treated with biofeedback procedures (c.f.,
Budzynski and Stoyva, 1973).

Since facial pain represents a problem for both physicians and dentists, emphasis is placed on discussing the
variety of problems seen in the clinic. Just as physicians
should know not to inject the temporomandibular joint,
dentists should know not to treat trigeminal neuralgia by
full mouth extraction. Dealing with the atypical facial
neuralgia patient offers students the opportunity to once
more examine the problems of psychogenic versus organic
pain and how to treat it.

The classes on the pharmacology of pain, survey for
the student the variety of pain control substances and their
methods of use. The student is made aware of the fact that
for chronic pain conditions we quickly run out of medications. The search for the non-addicting pain-killer is
still on.

The neurosurgical approach to pain control reviews the
different types of procedures available, their effectiveness as well as their many possible complications. Here,
too the student can readily see that although surgery has
a place in pain control, it is quite limited.

                           CONCLUDING REMARKS

Although the American Dental Association has published
guidelines on a comprehensive program of pain control
(1972), the emphasis is almost completely pharmacological.
"Human behavior and psychologic aspects of pain and appre-
hension" are mentioned but only as background to the use
of other techniques. Nowhere are the behavioral possibilities fully developed.

I have searched through the Journal of Medical Education and the Journal of Dental Education for the past four
years. Aside from the just mentioned ADA guidelines or a

clerkship in anesthesiology, there is almost no mention of
formalized teaching of comprehensive pain control. Given
the central importance of this area, it seems to be a void
in our current curricula.

The course just described is by no means complete by
itself. It should be expanded especially during clinical
training. However, as many students have written in their
course evaluations it is the only place where they can
formally learn behavioral techniques as part of a more
comprehensive view of pain control.

REFERENCES

American Dental Association, Council on Dental Education.
Guidelines for teaching the comprehensive control of
pain and anxiety in dentistry. Journal of Dental Educa-
tion, 1972, XXXVI, 62-67.
Bandura, A., Principles of behavior modification. New York:
Holt, Rinehart and Winston, 1969.
Beecher, H.K. Pain: one mystery solved. Science, 1966, 151,
840-841.
Beecher, H.K. The placebo effect as a non-specific force
surrounding disease and the treatment of disease. In R.
Janzen, et al (Eds.) Pain: basic principles, pharmacology,
therapy. Stuttgart, Germany: Georg Thieme, 1972, 175-180.
Blitz, B. and Dinnerstein, A.J. Role of attentional focus
in pain perception: manipulation of response to noxious
stimulation by instructions. Journal of Abnormal Psychology, 1971, 77, 42-45.
Budzynski, T. and Stoyva, J. Biofeedback techniques in
behavior therapy. In D. Shapiro et al (Eds.) Biofeedback and self-control 1972. Chicago: Aldine, 1973,
Chapter 23.
Cohen, F. and Lazarus, R.S. Active coping processes, coping dispositions, and recovery from surgery. Psychoso-
matic Medicine, 1973, 35, 375-389.
Craig, K.D. and Weiss, S.M., Vicarious influences on pain-
threshold determinations. Journal of Personality and
Social Psychology, 1971, 19, 53-59.
Dalessio, D.J. Wolff's headache and other head pain. New
York: Oxford University Press, 1972, 3rd edition.
Egbert, L.D., Battit, G.E., Welch, C.E. and Bartlett, M.D.
Reduction of postoperative pain by encouragement and
instruction of patients. The New England Journal of
Medicine, 1964, 270, 825-827.

M. WEISENBERG

Fordyce, W.E., Fowler, R.S., Lehman, J.F., DeLateur, B.
  Some implications of learning in problems of chronic
  pain. Journal of Chronic Diseases, 1968, 21, 179-190.
Geldard, F.A., The human senses. New York, John Wiley and
  Sons, 1972.
Gordon, W.H. Why people go to quacks. Proceeding Third
  National Congress on Medical Quackery, Chicago, American
  Medical Association, 1966.
Hardy, J.D., Wolff, H.G., and Goodell, H., Pain sensations
  and reactions. New York: Hafner, 1952.
Hartland, J. Medical and dental hypnosis. London, England:
  Baillere, Tindall, and Cassell, 1971.
Hilgard, E.R., A neodissociation interpretation of pain
  reduction in hypnosis. Psychological Review, 1973, 80,
  396-411.
Jacobson, E. Progressive relaxation. Chicago, Illinois:
  University of Chicago Press, 1938.
Janis, I.L. Psychological stress. New York: John Wiley
  and Sons. 1958.
Johnson, J.E. Effects of accurate expectations about sensa-
  tions on the sensory and distress components of pain.
  Journal of Personality and Social Psychology, 1973, 27,
  261-275.
Johnson, J.E. and Leventhal, H. Effects of accurate expectations and behavioral instructions on reactions during
  a noxious medical examination. Journal of Personality
  and Social Psychology, 1974, 29, 710-718.
Kenshalo, D.R., The cutaneous senses, In J.W. Kling and
  L.A. Riggs (Eds.), Woodworth and Schlossberg's experimental psychology. New York: Holt, Rinehart and Winston,
  1971.
Linn, E.L., Role behaviors in two dental clinics: a trial
  of Nadel's criterea. Human Organization, 1967, 26,
  141-148.
Melzack, R. The puzzle of pain. New York: Basic Books,
  1973.
Melzack, R. and Wall, P.D., Psychophysiology of pain. The
  International Anesthesiology Clinics, 1970, 8, 3-34.
Miller, N.E., Barber, T.X., DiCara, L.V., Kamiya, J.,
  Shapiro, D., and Stoyva, J. Biofeedback and self-control
  1973. Chicago: Aldine, 1974.
Mountcastle, V.B., Pain and temperature sensibilities. In
  V.B. Mountcastle, (Ed.) Medical physiology, Saint Louis:
  C.V. Mosby, 1974.

Neufeld, R.W.J. and Davidson, P.O. The effects of vicarious and cognitive rehearsal on pain tolerance. Journal of Psychosomatic Research, 1971, 15, 329-335.

Pilowsky, I. and Bond, M.R. Pain and its management in malignant disease. Psychosomatic Medicine, 1969, XXXI, 400-404.

Schurmann, K. Surgical treatment: fundamental principles of the surgical treatment of pain. In R. Janzen et al (Eds.). Pain: basic principles, pharmacology, therapy, Stuttgart, Germany: Georg Thieme, 1972, 181-193.

Spear, F.G. Pain in psychiatric patients. Journal of Psychosomatic Research, 1967, 11, 187-193.

Staub, E., Tursky, B., Schwartz, G.E., Self-control and predictability: their effects on reactions to aversive stimulation. Journal of Personality and Social Psychology, 1971, 18, 157-162.

Sternbach, R.A. Pain: a psychophysiological analysis. New York: Academic Press, 1968.

Sternbach, R.A. Pain patients: traits and treatment. New York: Academic Press, 1974.

Thompson, K.F., The role of suggestion in pain and anxiety. In C.R. Bennett (Ed.), Conscious sedation in dental practice. St. Louis, Missouri: C.V. Mosby, 1974.

Weisenberg, M. Cultural and racial reactions to pain.   In M. Weisenberg (Ed.) The control of pain. New York: Psychological Dimensions, Inc., 1976, Chapter 5.

Wolpe, J. The practice of behavior therapy. New York: Pergamon, 1973.

Zimbardo, P.G., Cohen, A.R., Weisenberg, M., Dworkin, L., and Firestone, I. Control of pain motivation by cognitive dissonance. Science, 1966, 151, 217-219.

APPENDIX (Sample Course Outline)

1974 Spring Elective

THE PERCEPTION AND CONTROL OF PAIN

Faculty: M. Weisenberg, Ph.D. (Chairman)
           L. Daniels, Ph.D., M. Feinstein, Ph.D.,
           H. Fiss, Ph.D., C. Loeser, M.D., G. Owens, M.D.,
           S. Woo, M.D.

This course will look at the basic dimensions of pain
from a social, psychological, physiological and pharmacological point of view. It is aimed at achieving an in-
depth view of pain perception that will stress the multidisciplinary nature of pain control in the therapeutic
situation. It is not going to be sufficient to examine the
issues of pain from the textbook alone. Laboratory sessions for the purpose of learning techniques such as
relaxation, hypnosis, use of biofeedback, etc., will be an
integral part of the course.

Course Requirements. Each student will be responsible
for presentations to the class in at least one of the areas
within the course syllabus. Each student will also be
responsible for developing a paper covering in depth an
area of pain that is of particular interest to the student.
These requirements will be discussed in greater detail in
class.

In addition to formal classes, students will be expected to take advantage of the opportunities available in
patient care settings.

Reading will be assigned from the following books:

1. Melzack, R. The Puzzle of Pain. New York: Basic
      Books, 1973.
2. Dalessio, D.J. Wolff's Headache and Other Head Pain.
      New York: Oxford University Press, 1972, 3rd edi-
      tion.
3. Sternbach, R.A. Pain: A Psychophysiological Analysis.
      New York: Academic Press, 1968.

4. Zborowski, M. <u>People in Pain</u>. San Francisco, Calif.:
       Jossey-Bass, 1969.
5. Soulairac, A. et al (Eds.) <u>Pain: Proceedings of the
       International Symposium on Pain, April 11-13, 1967</u>.
       New York: Academic Press, 1968.
6. Janzen, R. et al (Eds.) <u>Pain: Basic Principles Pharma-
       cology Therapy</u>. Stuttgart: Georg Thieme Verlag,
       1972.

For the study of hypnosis, readings will be recommended
from the following books:

1. Erickson, M.H., Hershman, S., and Secter, I.I. <u>The
       Practical Application of Medical and Dental Hypnosis</u>.
       New York: The Julian Press, 1961.
2. Fross, G.H. <u>Handbook of Hypnotic Techniques</u>. Irving-
       ton, N.J.: Power Publishers, 1966.
3. Hartland, J. <u>Medical and Dental Hypnosis</u>. London:
       Bailliere, Tindall, and Cassell, 1966 or 1971 Second
       Edition.

Class Schedule and Topics (9:00 - 12:00)

Monday,   May 6   Film: "Pain: Where Does It Hurt
                        Most?" Dr. M. Weisenberg
                        Neuroanatomical Theories of Pain, Dr.
                        C. Loeser

Wednesday,   May 8   Laboratory: Introduction to Hypnosis,
                        Dr. M. Weisenberg, Dr. L. Daniels
                        Techniques of Measuring Pain, Dr. M.
                        Weisenberg

Friday,   May 10   Laboratory: Eye-Roll Technique, Dr.
                        M. Weisenberg, Dr. L. Daniels
                        Reactions to Pain: Perceptual and
                        Cognitive Factors, Dr. M. Weisenberg

Monday,   May 13   Laboratory: Achieving Analgesia with
                        Hypnosis, Dr. M. Weisenberg, Dr. L.
                        Daniels
                        Reactions to Pain: Psychiatric Con-
                        siderations, Dr. H. Fiss

Wednesday,   May 15   Laboratory: Use of Relaxation (Intro-
                        duction) Dr. M. Weisenberg
                        Stress, Anxiety and Pain, Dr. M.
                        Weisenberg

Thursday,   May 16   Laboratory: Introduction to Biofeed-
                        back, Dr. M. Weisenberg
                        Facial Pain, Dr. M. Weisenberg

Monday,   May 20   Laboratory: Biofeedback (Continued)
                        Dr. M. Weisenberg
                        Headache Pain, Dr. M. Weisenberg

Tuesday,   May 21   Laboratory: To Be Announced
                        Anesthesia Techniques, Dr. S. Woo

Wednesday,   May 22   Laboratory: To Be Announced
                        The Pharmacology of Analgesia, Dr. M.
                        Feinstein

Friday,   May 24   Laboratory: To Be Announced
                        The Surgical Relief of Pain, Dr. G.
                        Owens

Wednesday,   May 29   Laboratory: Symptom Removal Through
                        Hypnosis, Dr. M. Weisenberg
                        Cultural Reactions to Pain, Dr. M.
                        Weisenberg

Thursday,   May 30   Acupuncture, Dr. M. Weisenberg

Monday, May 6

   9-10   Introduction - Film "Pain: Where Does It Hurt
           Most?" Dr. M. Weisenberg
   10-12   Neuroanatomical Theories of Pain, Dr. C. Loeser

           Truex and Carpenter. Human Neuroanatomy. Wil-
              liam and Wilkins, 1969, 265-269, 364-371,
              470-472, 558-562.
           Casey, K.L. Pain - A current view of neural
              mechanisms. American Scientist, 1973, 61,
              194-200.
           Melzack, R. and Wall, P.D. Pain mechanisms:
              A new theory. Science, 1965, 150, 971-979.

Wall, P.D. and Dubner, R. Annual Review of
Physiology, 1972, 34, 325-326.
DeJong, R. Report on international symposium
on pain. Anesthesia, 1973, 39, 662-664.

Wednesday, May 8

9-10   Introduction to Hypnosis, Dr. M. Weisenberg,
Dr. L. Daniels

Weitzenhoffer, A.M. and Hilgard, E.R. Stanford
Hypnotic Susceptibility Scale. Palo Alto,
California: Consulting Psychologists Press,
1959.
Erickson, et al., Chapter 4 or Fross, Chapter
IV, or Hartland, Chapters 4-7.
Jacoby, J.D. Practical suggestions for dentists
working with the patient in a trance. The
American Journal of Clinical Hypnosis, 1967,
X, 39-43.

10-12   Techniques of Measuring Pain, Dr. M. Weisenberg

Hardy, J., Wolff, H.G., and Goodell, H. Pain
Sensations and Reactions. New York: Hafner
Publishing Co., 1967, Chapter III.
Beecher, H.K. Quantification of subjective
pain experience. Proceedings of the American Psychopathological Association, 1963,
53, 111-128.
Bloomfield, S.S. and Hurwitz, H.N. Tourniquet
and episiotomy pain as test models for
aspirin-like analgesics. The Journal of
Clinical Pharmacology, 1970, 10, 361-369.
Forgione, A.G. and Barber, T.X. A strain gauge
pain stimulator. Psychophysiology, 1971, 8,
102-106.
Kast, E.C. Clinical measurement of pain.
Medical Clinics of North America, 1968, 52,
23-32.
Tursky, B. and Watson, P.D. Controlled physical and subjective intensities of electric
shock. Psychophysiology, 1964, 1, 151-162.

Friday, May 10

    9-10   Laboratory: The Eye-Roll Technique, Dr. M.
                Weisenberg, Dr. L. Daniels

                Spiegel, H. An eye-roll test for hypnotiza-
                   bility. The American Journal of Clinical
                   Hypnosis, 1972, 15, 25-28.
                Spiegel, H. and Bridger, A.A. A Manual for
                   Hypnotic Induction Profile. New York: Soni
                   Medica, 1970.

   10-12   Perceptual and Cognitive Factors, Dr. M.
                Weisenberg

                Melzack, Chapters 1-4
                Sternbach, Chapter V
                Zimbardo, P.G., Cohen, A., Weisenberg, M.,
                 Dworkin, L., and Firestone, I. Control of
                 pain motivation by cognitive dissonance,
                 Science, 1966, 151, 217-219.
                Fordyce, W.E., Fowler, R.S., Lehmann, J.F. and
                 DeLateur, B. Some implications of learning
                 in problems of chronic pain. Journal of
                 Chronic Diseases, 1968, 21, 179-190.
                Craig, K.D. and Weiss, S.M. Verbal reports of
                 pain without noxious stimulation. Percep-
                 tual and Motor Skills, 1972, 34, 943-948.

Monday, May 13

    9-10   Laboratory: Analgesia Through Hypnosis. Dr.
                M. Weisenberg, Dr. L. Daniels

                Hartland, Chapter 12
                Erickson, M.H. The interspersal hypnotic tech-
                 nique for symptom correction and pain control.
                 The American Journal of Clinical Hypnosis,
                 1966, VIII, 198-209.
                Sacerdote, P. Theory and practice of pain
                 control in malignancy and other protracted
                 or recurring painful illnesses. The Inter-
                 national Journal of Clinical and Experi-
                 mental Hypnosis, XVIII, 160-180.

10-12   Psychiatric Considerations, Dr. Fiss

Szasz, T.S. Language and Pain in S. Arieti
    (Ed.) American Handbook of Psychiatry,
    Basic Books, 1966, Vol. 1, Chapter 49.
Case History (To be handed out)
Soulairac 93-113

Wednesday, May 15

9-10   Laboratory: Introduction to Relaxation, Dr. M.
         Weisenberg

Wolpe, J. The Practice of Behavior Therapy.
    New York: Pergamon Press, 1969, 100-107.
Bonica, J.J. Principles and Practice of
    Obstetric Analgesia and Anesthesia. Phila-
    delphia: F.A. Davis, 1967, Vol. 1, Chapters
    45-47.
Bernstein, D.A. and Bokovec, T.D. Progressive
    Relaxation Training. Champaign, Ill.: Re-
    search Press, 1973.

10-12   Stress, Anxiety and Pain, Dr. M. Weisenberg

Sternbach, Chapter IV
Weisenberg, M., Kreindler, M.L., Schachat, R.,
    and Werboff, J. Pain: Anxiety and attitudes
    in Black, White and Puerto Rican patients,
    Psychosomatic Medicine, 1974 in press.
Baldwin, D.C. An investigation of psychologi-
    cal and behavioral responses to dental ex-
    traction in children. Journal of Dental
    Research, 1966, 45, 1637-1651.
Abram, H.S. and Gill, B.F. Predictions of
    postoperative psychiatric complications.
    The New England Journal of Medicine, 1961,
    265, 1123-1128.
Egbert, L.D., Battit, G.E., Welch, C.E. and
    Bartlett, M.K. Reduction of postoperative
    pain by encouragement and instruction of
    patients. The New England Journal of Medi-
    cine, 1964, 270, 825-827.

Johnson, J.E., Dabbs, J.M., and Leventhal, H.
Psychosocial factors in the welfare of
surgical patients. Nursing Research, 1970,
19, 18-29.
Janis, I.C. Some implications of recent research on the dynamics of fear and stress
tolerance. Social Psychiatry, 1969, XLVII,
86-100.
Lazarus, R.S., Opton, E.M., Nomikos, M.S., and
Rankin, N.O. The principle of short-cir-
cuiting of threat: further evidence. Journal of Personality, 1965, 33, 622-635.

Thursday, May 16

9-10   Laboratory: Introduction to Biofeedback, Dr.
M. Weisenberg

Budzynski, T. and Stoyva, J. Biofeedback techniques in behavior therapy, in D. Shapiro
et al (Eds.) Biofeedback and Self-Control
1972. Chicago: Aldine, 1973, Chapter 33.

10-12   Facial Pain, Dr. M. Weisenberg

Dalessio, Chapters 15, 16
Ingle, J.I. Endodontics. Philadelphia: Lea
and Febinger, 1965, Chapter 11.
Greene, C.S. A survey of current professional
concepts and opinions about the myofacial
pain-dysfunction syndrome. JADA, 1973, 86,
128-136.
Laskin, D.M. Etiology of the pain-dysfunction
syndrome. JADA, 1969, 79, 147-153.

Monday, May 20

9-10   Laboratory: Biofeedback (Continued), Dr. M.
Weisenberg

Budzynski, T. and Stoyva, J. An electromyo-
graphic feedback technique for teaching
voluntary relaxation of the masseter muscle.
Journal of Dental Research, 1973, 52, 116-
119.

10-12   Headache Pain

         Dalessio, Chapter 8, 228-230; Chapters 11, 12

Tuesday, May 21

9-10   Laboratory: Practice of Hypnotic Induction and
         Deepening, Dr. M. Weisenberg, Dr. L. Daniels

         Review relevant sections in Hartland, Fross or
         Erickson

10-12   Anesthesia Techniques, Dr. S. Woo

         Covino, B.G. Local anesthesia. NEJM, 1972, 286,
         975-983, 1035-1042.
         Moore, D.C. and Bridenbaugh, L.D. Spinal
         (subarachnoid) block. JAMA, 1966, 195, 907-
         912.
         Shealy, C.N., Taslitz, N., Mortimer, J.T., and
         Becker, D.P. Electrical inhibition of pain.
         Anesth. Analg. Curr. Res., 1967, 46, 299-305.
         Lloyd, J.W., Hughes, J.T., and Davies-Jones,
         G.A.B. Relief of severe intractable pain by
         barbotage of cerebro-spinal fluid. Lancet,
         1972, 1, 354-355.

Wednesday, May 22

9-10   Laboratory: To Be Announced

10-12   The Pharmacology of Analgesia, Dr. M. Feinstein

         Eddy, N.B. and May, E.L. The search for a bet-
         ter analgesic. Science, 1973, 181, 407-414.
         Lim, R.K.S. and Guzman, F. Manifestations of
         pain in analgesic evaluation in animals and
         man. In Pain, Proc. Intl. Sympos. on Pain,
         (Eds.) Soulairac, Cahn and Charpentier,
         Academic Press, N.Y. 1968, 119-152.
         Beecher, H.K. The measurement of pain in man.
         ibid. 201-213.
         Eckenhoff, J.E. and Oech, S.R. The effects of
         narcotics and antagonists upon respiration
         and circulation in man. Clin. Pharmac. Ther.
         1960, 1, 483-524.

Smith, G.M., Lowenstein, E., Hubbard, J.H., and
    Beecher, H.K. Experimental pain produced by
    the submaximum effort tourniquet technique:
    further evidence of validity. J. Pharmac.
    Exp. Ther., 1968, 163, 468-474.
Wolff, B.B., Kantor, T.G., Jarvik, M.E., and
    Laska, E. Response of experimental pain to
    analgesic drugs. I. Morphine, aspirin, and
    placebo. Clin. Pharmac. Ther., 1966, 7, 224-
    238.
    Response of experimental pain to analgesic
    drugs. III. Codeine, aspirin, secobarbital
    and placebo. ibid., 1969, 10, 217-228.
Jasinski, D.R., Martin, W.R., and Sapira, J.D.
    Antagonism of the subjective, behavioral,
    pupillary and respiratory depressant effects
    of cycazacine by naloxone. Clin. Pharmac.
    Ther., 1968, 9, 215-222.
Guzman, F. and Lim, R.K.S. The mechanism of
    action of the non-narcotic analgesics. Med.
    Clinics of North America, 1968, 52, 3-14.
Paton, W.D.M. In Scientific basis of drug de-
    pendence. (Ed.) H. Steinberg, London:
    Churchill, 31.
Collier, H.O.J. A general theory of the genesis
    of drug dependence by induction of receptors.
    Nature, 1965, 205, 181-182.
Kosterlitz, H.W. and Watt, A.J. Brit. J. Phar-
    macol., 1968, 33, 266.

Friday, May 24

   9-11   The Surgical Relief of Pain, Dr. G. Owens

          Janzen, 181-222.

Wednesday, May 29

   9-10   Laboratory: Symptom Removal Through Hypnosis,
          Dr. M. Weisenberg, Dr. L. Daniels

          Read relevant sections of Erickson or Hartland
          on symptom removal.

  10-12   Cultural Reactions to Pain, Dr. M. Weisenberg

Zborowski, M. <u>People in Pain</u>. San Francisco:
    Jossey-Boss, 1969.
Weisenberg, M. Cultural and racial reactions to
    pain. Paper deliver to AAAS, February, 1974.
Wolff, B.B. and Langley, S. Cultural factors
    and the response to pain: A review. <u>Ameri-
    can Anthropologist</u>, 1968, 70, 494-501.

Thursday, May 30

   9-12   Acupuncture, Dr. M. Weisenberg

   9-10   Films on acupuncture

10-12   Discussion
Van Nghi, N., Fisch, G., and Kao, J. An intro-
    duction to classical acupuncture. <u>American
    Journal of Chinese Medicine</u>, 1973, 1, 75-83.
Melzack, R. How acupuncture can block pain.
    <u>Impact of Science on Society</u>, 1973, 65-75.
Chaves, J.F. and Barber, T.X. Acupuncture
    analgesia: six factors to help to explain
    the efficacy of acupuncture in attenuating
    surgical pain. <u>Human Behavior</u>, Los Angeles:
    Manson Western Corp., 1973.
Melzack, Chapters 6, 7.

PAIN: PAST, PRESENT, AND FUTURE*

Ronald Melzack

McGill University

Montreal, Quebec, Canada

The recent descriptions of major surgery carried out in China with "acupuncture analgesia" have evoked enormous excitement in Western countries. There are frequent descriptions and evaluations of the phenomenon in the popular press. Many Western governments--particularly the United States, Canada, and Britain--have received large quantities of mail demanding close examination and evaluation of this method of pain control. Administrative officials who never gave pain research a moment's thought are now in the position of having to make decisions about it. "Acupuncture analgesia," whatever the underlying mechanisms turn out to be, may have the same catalytic impact on pain research in the United States that the Russian Sputnik had on the U.S. space program. Certainly it means that pain has become a major research problem that involves widespread segments of the medical and biological research community. It will undoubtedly receive increasing attention and, therefore, will generate increasing demands for financial support.

THE PAST

Curiosity about acupuncture analgesia is only part of a major rise in interest and research in pain mechanisms in recent years. Until the last five years or so, pain was a

---

* This paper is based on a report prepared for: Committee on Psychological Processes, National Institute of Mental Health, Mental Health Intramural Research Program.

relatively "minor" research topic. In most textbooks in
physiology, psychology, anatomy, even neurology, it was
lumped with smell, taste, touch, and the other "minor senses." It received a paragraph or two, and was dismissed as
either a problem that was solved long ago or, less often,
as one that is hopelessly bogged down in an esoteric argu-
ment between two opposing theories (specificity and pattern
theories). Laboratory research was minimal, with perhaps a
dozen papers per year that dealt directly with pain mechanisms. (I am excluding, for the moment, pharmacological research on analgesic and anesthetic agents--an important
field, but one which has not been aimed at revealing the
nature of pain mechanisms.)

There have been occasional periods of considerable research activity on pain, particularly in the 1940's and due
almost entirely to the work of Drs. Hardy, Wolff, and Goodell. It was sound, respectable work--an attempt to quantify
pain using psychophysical methods--but in retrospect is seen
to have led to a dead-end. It generated research that re-
volved around the conceptual notion that pain was trans-
mitted through a fixed-gain system and characteristically
had a one-to-one relationship to stimulus intensity. Some
new, important ideas were expressed in the book that summarized the work--ideas which indicated a greater plasticity
in neural processes related to pain--but these were largely
lost in the overall psychophysical thrust of the book (Hardy,
Wolff, and Goodell, 1952).

For the most part, Hardy, Wolff, and Goodell's book,
published in 1952, together with Sweet's chapter on Pain in
the Handbook of Physiology (1959), led to the general consensus that the problem of pain was largely solved. The
traditional theory of pain--specificity theory--was taught
in most medical schools as gospel-truth, not a theory proposed in 1895. Pain was considered to be a specific sensory
system, with pain receptors and fibers that projected
through a specific pain pathway to a pain center in the
brain. The pain fibers were identified as A-delta and C
fibers, the pain receptors as free nerve endings, and the
spinothalamic tract was labelled as the pain pathway. All
that seemed to remain was to identify the pain center in the
brain. The status of the field was hardly one that would
entice the bright graduate student in search of a research
problem.

Despite the prestige given to specificity theory by eminent neurosurgeons, neurologists, and physiologists, there were a few important sceptics. W. K. Livingston wrote an important book on pain mechanisms in 1943 which dealt with pain phenomena (such as phantom limb pain and causalgia) that defied explanation in terms of specificity theory, and he proposed a new conceptual approach. The work was given lip-service by many writers, but was largely ignored. A few other excellent clinical observers described pain syndromes and failures of surgery for pain that demanded a re-evaluation of the field, but they had relatively little impact on the field. Nevertheless, this literature grew slowly until powerful, convincing arguments against specificity theory could be presented in the 1960's. A major source of evidence against specificity theory was H. K. Beecher's work, summarized in a book in 1959, which dealt with placebo responses and other important observations on the frequent absence of one-to-one relationships between stimulus and perception in pain (such as the denial by soldiers wounded in battle that they feel pain). Beecher, however, avoided a confrontation with specificity theory by suggesting that pain was a primary (specific) sensation and that variations in pain experience represented differing reactions to pain rather than pain itself. Investigators outside the U. S. also began to seriously undermine specificity theory. Noordenbos (1959) in Holland, and Weddell (1955) in England (both greatly influenced by W. K. Livingston) produced theoretical speculations as well as anatomical evidence that pointed toward pattern theory, a view proposing greater plasticity in perceptual processes.

In the late 1950's and early 1960's, it is now apparent, the field was in ferment. Powerful evidence against specificity theory had accumulated, but no convincing alternative theory was available to take its place. (Pattern theory was too vague and encountered difficulties that do not require analysis here.) The evidence came from three fields:

1. Clinical observations of phantom limb pain, causalgia, the neuralgias, and so forth, which could not be cured by conventional neurosurgical approaches, and which indicated the need for new conceptual and theoretical orientations.

2. Psychological observations that pain thresholds

varied as a function of culture, early experience, attention, the meaning of the situation
and other variables. Observations were made
with both human and animal subjects. The evidence, taken together, indicated that these
psychological factors play a powerful role in
determining the presence or absence of pain,
or the level of perceived pain in given situations.

3. Neurophysiological and anatomical studies that
indicated that fibers and cells in the somatic
sensory projection system could not always be
neatly categorized as belonging to warmth, cold,
touch or pain. Physiological evidence against
the theory of four specific modalities of cutaneous sensation was so convincing that the theory
became increasingly untenable.

In 1965, Melzack and Wall formulated a new theory of
pain that has gained increasing recognition. It is clear
that the theory rode in on a "zeitgeist," and both men were
astonished at its wide acceptance. The theory, basically,
proposes that a gate-like mechanism exists in the somatic
transmission system so that pain signals can be modulated
before they evoke perception and response. The gate can be
opened or closed by variable amounts, depending on factors
such as the relative activity in large and small peripheral
fibers, and various psychological processes such as attention and prior experience. By proposing a variable gate,
it became possible to attempt to close the gate by various
manipulations (which will be described below).

Whether the particular explanatory mechanisms proposed
by Melzack and Wall are correct or not, the theory has stimulated a large amount of research. The fact that techniques
to control pain have derived from the theory has undoubtedly
also been extremely important in its effect on the field.

DIRECTIONS FOR THE IMMEDIATE FUTURE

The emphasis on pain as a specific modality of cutaneous sensation was characterized, in past years, by two
major methods of approach: 1) lesions of transmission

pathways and related areas in the CNS, and 2) psychophysical
studies that sought precise, mathematical relationships between stimulus and sensation. The exciting, new directions,
then, are those that move away from the earlier approaches.

a. Stimulation Techniques

        In contrast to methods of making destructive, irre-
versible lesions in the central nervous system, or section-
ing peripheral nerves and dorsal roots, there has recently
been a sharp movement toward a more "physiological" approach.
In the CNS, attempts have been made to diminish pain by
stimulation of brain structures. In particular, work by
Reynolds (1969) and by Mayer and Liebeskind (1974) has indicated that electrical stimulation of midbrain structures
in rats produces a marked analgesia in portions of the body.
The rats were strikingly less responsive to intense, noxious stimulation such as pinch, freezing cold or shock.
Reynolds was even able to carry out major surgical operations
on rats which were stimulated in parts of the brainstem.
Mayer and Liebeskind were able to show that the stimulation
could be relatively specific, affecting a half or quadrant
of the body. Furthermore, they showed that the sites that
produced analgesia were also effective for self-stimulation.
There is evidence that these effects can be obtained in cats
and man but the best documented studies are those with the
rat. These analgesic effects produced by brain stimulation
are presumably due to activation of descending or ascending
inhibitory systems, but other mechanisms can be visualized
as well. These findings represent a major breakthrough,
and many laboratories are beginning to investigate the phenomenon in depth.

        Electrical stimulation of peripheral nerves, to selec-
tively activate large fibers, is another exciting approach
which has produced striking relief of pain in patients who
have undergone surgical operations (such as rhizotomy or
cordotomy) without being helped. The stimulation usually
produces a tingling feeling and diminution of pain. Pain
may be abolished for many hours after cessation of stimulation. An intense, brief, painful stimulation may produce
even more prolonged, dramatic relief. Little is known about
the effect; again, it is an exciting research area.

Finally, direct stimulation of the skin by vibration, heat, cold, etc. is another effective method. It is related to the "counter-irritation" methods of folk-medicine. It may also be related to acupuncture as well as to observations that a momentary pain produced at one site (eg., the back) can abolish pain at another site (such as phantom limb pain). Some interesting research on this problem has begun and more is certain to follow.

b. Spatial Aspects of Pain

The fact that stimulation at one site on the body can affect pain at a distant site has long been known. The evidence indicates that more is involved than mere distraction or suggestion. There is, therefore, increasing interest in mechanisms that could underlie such effects. The substantia gelatinosa in the spinal cord could, theoretically, mediate such effects. Higher, brainstem mechanisms could also do so. These kinds of integrative mechanisms are of major importance in understanding pain.

c. Temporal Aspects of Pain

It was noted above that pain relief often outlasts electrical or other stimulation. Similarly, phantom limb pain can be abolished for weeks or months by a temporary anesthetic block. Furthermore, a temporary noxious stimulus may produce prolonged, persistent pain that can only be attributed to something like a memory trace in the CNS, rather than local irritation. These temporal properties have received little attention but merit much more. It is an important field for investigation.

d. Psychological Effects on Pain

It is well known that suggestion, hypnosis, distraction and other psychological variables can have a dramatic effect on pain. The evidence on this is convincing. Yet, there have been few attempts to utilitze these techniques in a concerted effort to relieve clinical pain. The number of workers in this field is increasing, however, and it represents an important new approach to pain. It could reveal a great deal about the basic mechanisms of pain.

e. Pharmacological Studies

A large number of chemists, pharmacologists and workers in related fields are in pursuit of new pharmacological agents to control pain. Much of this work is of a pedestrian, hit-and-miss sort. Sometimes, however, important breakthroughs occur. The discovery that carbamazepine (Tegretol) can cure <u>tic douleureux</u> and some other pain states has important theoretical implications. It is essentially an anti-convulsive drug, and appears to help pain in which muscle spasms are part of the whole picture. The effect of the drug is presumably on the CNS, however, and it throws light on the kinds of abnormal neural activities that may be involved in pain.

Perhaps the most exciting breakthrough is the discovery that the analgesia-producing areas in the brainstem are serotonergic. Furthermore, they appear to represent a major site of action of morphine. There is even evidence of endogenous production of morphine in these areas. These obserations are certain to have a profound effect on future research on the pharmacology of pain.

f. Clinical Observations

It is clear that first-rate clinical observation can have a powerful impact on any biological field. It was the thoughtful clinical observer, such as W. K. Livingston in the U. S. and Noordenbos in Holland, that set the stage for the "revolution" in pain concepts. It follows from this that we need more clinical neurologists trained to look for the unusual and not to be afraid to report observations that do not fit accepted medical teaching. In the case of pain, such people could be trained specifically in Pain Clinics.

PATTERN OF DEVELOPMENT IN THE FIELD

The pattern of development of pain research in recent years provides an almost perfect illustration of Conant's

(1947) and Kuhn's (1962) views of the development of science.
There is a slow, un-remarkable accumulation of data in the
field, some of it contradictory to the prevailing theory.
After a while, there is ferment and controversy in the field.
Then a new theory is proposed that integrates both old and
new facts and leads to a sudden growth of interest and new
research in the field. This is precisely what has happened
in pain research in recent years. The growth of interest
in the field has been enormous, and research will probably
continue to flourish at this high level for several decades.

SIGNIFICANT PROBLEMS AND QUESTIONS

Techniques for measuring pain in man and animals are
still relatively primitive. There is an urgent need to cope
with this problem. On the human side, such methods of measurement as using fractions or numbers to represent changes
in pain intensity reveal only one dimension of pain. Pain,
however, is multi-dimensional. It has obvious temporal and
spatial properties as well as a variety of other sensory
and affective dimensions. Melzack and Torgerson (1971) have
made a start toward revealing the dimensions, and Melzack
has devised a pain questionnaire to specify and quantify
them in clinical settings. Hopefully, this approach will
broaden the possibility of pain research using human subjects
who are already in pain. Much more work is needed here.

In animals, the tests are mostly artificial, and I believe they result in the loss of valuable data, such as in
the pharmacological field. The hot-plate test, and the
tail-flick test are generally threshold tests. Electric
shock is also usually employed at threshold level. Yet,
there is convincing evidence that procedures that affect
pain at intense levels may have little or no effect on pain
at threshold levels. The titration technique, for example,
has missed finding the analgesic properties of midbrain
stimulation. Stimulation appears to produce analgesia to
intense, noxious stimulation, but seems to lower threshold
to shock--a seemingly anomalous finding, but in fact, not
entirely surprising. New techniques for pain research with
animals are urgently needed.

This raises an important question. Investigators are
reluctant to use frankly painful stimuli in animal studies.

They evoke the scorn of their colleagues, of journal editors, and anti-vivisectionists. Yet, I know of no other way to study pain than to use painful stimuli. Naturally, the investigator must use those stimuli that cause least pain for a given problem under study, and stimuli that do not produce pain that outlasts stimulation. This is a serious ethical problem for each individual investigator and one that raises the relationship of the scientist to his society. A given investigator who has seen terrible human suffering may develop a set of ethical priorities that permit him to cause pain in animals (if he is convinced that his work will ultimately lead to diminished suffering in man and animals at a later time). However, it is often hard to convince the layman of this reasoning, and the problem needs to be considered as a special case in studies using animals in research. Pain cannot be studied in the anesthetized animal, or by using stimuli which are not painful. Both methods mis-lead rather than enlighten. (Having personally been the object of attacks by the anti-vivisectionist press, I know how much it "hurts" to be considered an evil, brutal sadist when my aims were, in my estimation, genuinely humanitarian.

A further important problem is our need for knowledge of specialization of function in the central nervous system. Wall and his colleagues, and others (eg., Wagman and Price, 1969; Spencer and April, 1970) have done much to reveal spinal cord mechanisms. We still have little information about the destinations of pain signals in the brainstem, thalamus, and cortex, and of the changes and interactions such signals must undergo. There have recently been some outstanding studies (eg., by Casey and his students, 1973), but far too few. The activities of the <u>brain</u> related to pain still present the major gap in our knowledge. Since stimulation techniques seem the most promising, we must recognize that such studies will require the invention of new techniques and the use of frankly painful stimuli.

FACTORS THAT RESTRAIN PROGRESS

The major restraining factor in pain research at present is the paucity of people in the field. The field is growing, but new people need to be attracted to the area. Pain is a potentially important field not only because it holds promise of relief of suffering, but because it can

serve as a focus par excellence to bring together investigators from widely diverging fields, and it is exceptional in
the degree to which clinical and experimental studies are
tied together. These ties in other fields (eg., memory,
language) have produced mutual enrichment (of, for example,
both psychology and neurology). Similar, perhaps greater,
enrichment can occur in the field of pain.

N.I.M.H.'s CONTRIBUTION

The contribution has obviously been enormous. All the
people involved in the major experimental and theoretical
advances in the field in the United States, Canada, and
Britain have received N.I.M.H. support. I do not know of a
major U. S. investigator of pain problems who has failed to
get N.I.M.H. support. The methods of evaluation and distribution of funds has worked in the past and will undoubtedly continue to work effectively. Because of the growth
of work in this field, however, and because of its clear
potential value to humanity, the field needs to be developed
to a far greater degree. New research on pain should be
actively encouraged and promoted by providing funds for
symposia, special meetings, trips by senior investigators
and students to active laboratories and hospitals, and so
forth. N.I.M.H. has already undertaken some of these activities. Much more is needed.

REFERENCES

Beecher, H.K. (1959) Measurement of Subjective Responses,
    Oxford University Press.
Casey, K.L. (1973) 'Pain: a current view of neural mech-
    anisms.' American Scientist, vol. 61, p. 194.
Conant, J.B. (1947) On Understanding Science. Yale Uni-
    versity Press.
Hardy, J.D., Wolff, H.G., and Goodell, H. (1952) Pain
    Sensations and Reactions, Williams and Wilkins.
Kuhn, T.S. (1962) The Structure of Scientific Revolutions.
    University of Chicago Press.
Livingston, W.K. (1943) Pain Mechanisms, MacMillan.

Mayer, D.J. and Liebeskind, J.C.   (1974)   'Pain reduction
    by focal electrical stimulation of the brain: an ana-
    tomical and behavioral analysis.'   Brain Research, vol.
    68, p. 73.
Melzack, R. and Torgerson, W.S.   (1971)   'On the language
    of pain.'   Anesthesiology, vol. 34, p. 50.
Melzack, R. and Wall, P.D.   (1965)   'Pain mechanisms: a new
    theory.'   Science, vol. 150, p. 971.
Noordenbos, W.   (1959)   Pain.   Elsevier Press.
Reynolds, D.V.   (1969)   'Surgery in the rat during electri-
    cal analgesia induced by focal brain stimulation.'   Sci-
    ence, vol. 164, p. 444.
Spencer, W.A. and April, R.S.   (1970)   'Plastic properties
    of monosynaptic pathways in mammals.'   in G. Horn and
    R. A. Hinde (eds.), Short-Term Changes in Neural Activity
    and Behaviour, Cambridge, University Press.
Sweet, W.H.   (1959)   'Pain'   Handbook of Physiology, vol. 1,
    p. 459.
Wagman, I.H. and Price, P.D.   (1969)   'Responses of dorsal
    horn cells of M. mulatta to cutaneous and sural nerve A
    and C fibre stimuli.'   J. Neurophysiol., vol. 32, p. 803.
Weddell, G.   (1955)   'Somesthesis and the chemical senses.'
    Annual Review of Psychol., vol. 6, p. 119.

PAIN IN PERIPHERAL NEUROPATHY RELATED TO SIZE AND RATE OF FIBER DEGENERATION

Peter James Dyck, E. H. Lambert, and
Peter O'Brien
Mayo Clinic and Mayo Foundation

Rochester, Minnesota

An understanding of the mechanisms underlying spontaneous painfulness in pheripheral neuropathy of man might provide an insight into mechanisms of pain in general. Pain in peripheral neuropathy is of several kinds. Spontaneous momentary sharp jabs of pain is one kind. A more prolonged and often phasic aching, burning, stinging discomfort is a second. Both types of pain may occur together. Pain may be described as superficial in the skin or deep or as both superficial and deep. It is generally appreciated by neurologists that pain in peripheral neuropathy is often associated with a decrease of cutaneous sensation, i.e. elevation of threshold of sensation. It has not been established whether pain is associated with a selective decrease or loss of one modality of sensation as compared to another, e.g. pain vs. touch-pressure sensation. When the raised threshold is exceeded, an external stimulus may result in a painful sensation which is excessive, of long duration and involving a greater territory than in healthy persons. Our own studies have shown that patients with selective and severe impairment of mechano-receptor function without impairment of pain sensation, as occurs for example in early Friedreich's Ataxia, had a decrease in amplitude only of the alpha potential and markedly decreased numbers especially of large diameter fibers of cutaneous nerves. Neuropathic pain was not a feature of this group of patients. Conversely, patients with relatively selective impairment

This investigation was supported in part by Research Grants NSO 5811, NSO 7541, AM2-2200, MDA-8 and Upton Fund.

of pain sensation, of thermal discrimination and of autonomic function, as occurs, for example in some cases of dominantly inherited amyloidosis and dominantly inherited sensory neuropathy, had a selective decrease in amplitude or absence of the Aδ and C potentials and on histologic evaluation had a marked decrease or absence of small myelinated and unmyelinated fibers. Not uncommonly pain was present in this group of patients.

These observations raised the possibility that pain in peripheral neuropathy is related to damage, or to the result of damage of pain fibers in Aδ and drC fiber groups. Since neurophathic pain was not present in all patients with disorders thought to have degeneration of Aδ and C fibers, other factors such as rate of degeneration might be playing a modifying role. Alternatively the hypothesis might be wrong--a view held by the proponents of the gate theory of pain.

To test whether pain in peripheral neuropathy is related to rate of degeneration of unmyelinated and small diameter myelinated fibers (populations containing pain fibers), we have evaluated the degree of pain, the rate of fiber degeneration, and the amplitudes of Aα and C potentials of excised sural nerve of 72 patients with peripheral neuropathy. Pain was graded from the patient's history: 1=no pain, 2=slight pain, 3=moderate pain, and 4=severe pain. The rate of fiber degeneration was estimated in two ways. The first was by judging the rapidity of nerve fiber degeneration by disease category. In the first group of diseases fibers degenerate rapidly to form linear rows of myelin break-down products. In the second group the fiber degeneration is much slower and fibers undergo an atrophic process which is different from the above. The diseases placed into the rapid and slow categories are shown in Table 1.

PAIN IN RAPID VS SLOWLY PROGRESSIVE DISORDERS

Pain occurred in 76 percent of patients in group 1 (the more rapid progression group) and in only 15 percent of patients in group 2 (the slow progression group). The difference is highly significant, suggesting that the rapidity of fiber degeneration is correlated with painfulness (see Table 2).

Table 1. Varieties of peripheral neuropathy and number of
patients with rapid and intermediate progression (group 1)
and with slow progression (group 2)

Group 1		Group 2	
Disease	N	Disease	N
Infl. Polyradiculoneurop.	10	HN-CMT	9
Amyloidosis	4	N-CMT	7
Arsenic	2	HN-DS	5
Hypothyroidism	2	FA	5
Necrotizing Angiopathy	1	HSN-I	4
Drug	1	HSN-II	4
Diabetic	1		
Multiple Myeloma	1		
Carcinoma	1		
Pernicious Anemia	1		
Alcohol	1		

The 13 patients in which the diagnosis was unknown are not
included here.

Next we evaluated pain and rate of fiber degeneration
as judged by the frequency of linear rows of myelin ovoids
and balls in teased fibers of sural nerve.

The frequency of linear rows of myelin ovoids and balls
in teased fiber preparations is an index of rate of fiber
degeneration. It is known that transected myelinated fibers
will undergo this change before their disappearance. Many
acute and subacute neuropathic processes result in this degenerative condition. In very chronic neuropathic processes
this degenerative condition is only rarely seen. A low rate
of this abnormality is seen in healthy nerves. As shown in
Table 3, the mean percent of fibers undergoing this kind of
degeneration increases with increasing severity of pain.
Because the number of patients with pain of severity 3 and
4 is small these results must be interpreted with caution.
The mean frequency of this degenerative condition in patients
without pain (group 1) and with pain (groups 2, 3, and 4)

Table 2. Painfulness and Rapidity of Progression of Disease

	Group 1	Group 2
No pain	(24%)	(85%)
Pain	(76%)	(15%)
Total	25 (100%)	34 (100%)
		p < .001

was 4.83 and 15.64 percent respectively (.01<p<.025 Mann-Whitney Rank Sum Test). We conclude, therefore, that pain in this series of patients with peripheral neuropathy is positively correlated with rate of degeneration of nerve fibers.

Unfortunately, the characteristics of linear rows of myelin ovoids and balls does not permit us to say with reliability whether a particular linear row represents the remains of a large or small myelinated fiber. From these results it is therefore not possible to say whether pain results from degeneration of large or small fibers

Using the amplitdues of Aα and C potentials as an index of the relative number of remaining large myelinated and of unmyelinated fibers in sural nerve, we compared the mean amplitudes of these potentials and the ratio between

Table 3. The frequency (percent) of linear rows of myelin ovoids in patients with varying degrees of pain

	Pain			
	1	2	3	4
n	24	15	3	2
Mean	4.83	9.13	25.37	49.80
SD	10.15	12.37	21.01	15.70

them in the group of patients with diseases with a rapid
progression as compared to those with slow progression. As
shown in Tables 4, 5, and 6 mean values of Aα and C potentials were not significantly different in the two groups.
The means of the ratio of Aα/C amplitudes of the two groups
were compared. Using the Mann-Whitney Rank Sum Test no
significant difference was found.

Comparisons of the mean amplitude of Aα and C potentials and of the ratio of Aα/C potentials for patients without pain as compared to patients with pain in only the
group with rapid progression (group 1) did not show a significant mean difference using the Mann-Whitney Rank Sum Test.
From this evaluation we cannot say, therefore, that the
rapidly progressive group has more pain because of a different number of large and of small fibers or of the ratio between them.

Next we tested whether painfulness irrespective of rate
of disease was related to the amplitudes of Aα and C potentials or to the ratio between them. Using regression analysis of amplitudes or of ratio of amplitudes on degree of
pain, no significant relationship was found.

In spite of our results, painfulness may still be due
to degeneration of pain fibers in Aδ or C fiber groups or
to the effect of such degeneration. Perhaps the association
is not clear because we are not able to directly determine
the rate of degeneration of pain fibers in Aδ or C groups.
Of small myelinated and unmyelinated fibers only a small
proportion are known, from single fiber neurophysiologic
studies, to be concerned with nociception.

Table 4. Mean Amplitudes of Aα and C potentials and rapidity of progression of neuropathy

	Group 1			Group 2			P
	Mean	SD	% of Control	Mean	SD	% of control	ns
Aα (mv)	0.4	0.6	19.3	0.2	0.3	13.3	ns
C (μv)	51.1	38.3	69.2	49.4	28.4	66.9	ns

Table 5. Aα and C potentials of patients with rapid
progression (group 1)

		Aα			C
	n	mv	% of controls	mv	% of controls
Alcoholic	1	0	0	41	56
Acute Infl.	3	.2	11	44	59
Chr. and Relap. Infl.	7	.3	17	77	100
B-12 deficiency	1	1.6	89	89	100
Dom. Inh. Amyl.	2	.4	22	6	8
Prim. Amyl.	2	.2	11	36	41
Carcinoma	1	1.3	72	88	100
Multiple myeloma	1	.4	22	4	5
Diabetes mellitus	1	2.0	100	87	100
Drug	1	.2	11	74	100
Necrotizing Angiopathy	1	.1	5	45	61
Arsenic	2	.1	5	21	28
Hypothyroidism	2	0	0	29	39
Unknown	13	.5	28	41	54

Table 6. Aα and C potentials of patients with slow
progression (Group 2)

		Aα			C
	n	mv	% of controls	mv	% of controls
HN-CMT	9	.1	6	45	61
N-CMT	7	.2	11	65	88
HN-DS	5	0	0	46	62
FA	5	.3	17	67	91
HSN-I	4	.2	11	44	59
HSN-II	4	0	0	19	25

In summary we have shown that painfulness in a group of patients with peripheral neuropathy of man is related to rapidity of progression of disease and to the rate of degeneration of cutaneous nerve fibers. Because nociceptive fibers occur with a low frequency in small myelinated and unmyelinated fibers and since they cannot be recognized by histologic examination it has not been possible to test directly whether pain in peripheral neuropathy is related to rate of degeneration of nociceptive fibers or as an after effect of such degeneration. The nearest approximation to such a test has been to try and relate pain to the amplitudes of Aα and C potentials or of ratios between them. These comparisons have not shown that painfulness is related to selective involvement of small or of large fibers or to the ratio of small to large fibers which remain. This evaluation, therefore, does not rule out the possibility that pain in peripheral neuropathy is due to the rate of degeneration of nociciptive fibers or due to aftereffect of such degeneration. Our present bias is that pain in peripheral neuropathy is related to the rate of degeneration of nociceptive fibers. This view is based on the observations that chronic neuropathies in which large myelinated fibers disappear selectively do not have pain. Other chronic neuropathies, such as hereditary sensory neuropathy, with both large and small fiber degeneration not infrequently have pain. Recently, Ohnishi and co-workers (1974) have described two patients with Fabry's disease with a selective loss of small spinal ganglion neurons without a loss of large ganglion neurons. Both patients had much limb pain. In our opinion, therefore, painfulness is more likely to be due to rate of degeneration of pain fibers in Aδ and C fiber groups than due to degeneration of afferent fibers in Aα group.

REFERENCE

Ohnishi, Akio and Dyck, Peter James: Loss of Small Peripheral Sensory Neurons in Fabry Disease: histologic and morphometric evaluation of cutaneous nerves, spinal ganglia and posterior columns. Arch. Neurol. 31:120-127, Aug. 1974.

A BEHAVIORAL ANIMAL MODEL FOR THE STUDY OF PAIN MECHANISMS IN PRIMATES

R. Dubner, R. E. Beitel, and F. J. Brown

National Institute of Dental Research

Bethesda, Maryland

Recent neurophysiological studies in primates have increased significantly our knowledge of neural pathways that play a role in pain sensation and reaction. In the peripheral nervous system, neural populations have been identified which respond exclusively to intense or noxious stimuli applied to the skin (Burgess & Perl, 1973). Similarly, some neurons in the spinal cord dorsal horn with axon projections to the thalamus respond only to tissue-threatening or tissue-damaging stimuli (Willis, Trevino, Coulter, and Maunz, 1974; Price and Mayer, 1975). However, the situation is complicated by the finding that many spinothalamic neurons have a wide dynamic response range to innocuous and noxious mechanical stimuli (Willis et al, 1974; Price and Mayer, 1975). What role do such neurons play in pain? Furthermore, all of these studies have been performed under general anesthesia or after surgical brain lesions, both of which alter ongoing and evoked central neuronal activity. For example, dorsal horn neurons activated by noxious mechanical stimulation in a spinalized cat do not respond to similar stimuli in a decerebrated animal (Brown, 1971). Other studies have shown that cold block of the cervical spinal cord in anesthetized cats results in a significant increase in the sensitivity of lumbar spinal cord dorsal horn neurons to noxious heat stimuli (Zimmermann and Handwerker, 1974). Since the responsivity of these neurons is dependent upon the waking state of the animal, only tentative conclusions can be drawn from such experiments about the functional role of different spinal cord populations in pain.

A promising experimental approach is one that combines

the behavioral assessment of pain in animals with an analysis of peripheral and central neural events related to various components of such behavior. This approach has been attempted in studies of the medial medullary reticular formation in the region of nucleus gigantocellularis (Casey, Keene, and Morrow, 1974). This nucleus is considered part of an ascending pathway to medial thalamic structures presumed to play a role in the affective and motivational component of the pain experience (Melzack and Casey, 1968). Neuronal activity in nucleus gigantocellularis produced by electrical stimulation of a cutaneous nerve correlated highly with escape behavior in awake cats (Casey et al, 1974). Electrical stimulation of the same brainstem region also elicited escape behavior.

Although behavioral animal models which utilize an operant escape response to electric shock as a measure of pain have been employed extensively by experimental psychologists (Campbell and Church, 1969), there are some drawbacks to pure negative reinforcement paradigms: 1) Thresholds determined by the frequency of escape represent only one point on a continuum of behavior to aversive stimuli, and one which can be dissociated from such behavior by central nervous system lesions (Manning and Vierck, 1973; Vierck, Hamilton, and Thornby, 1971); 2) Electrical stimulation is an unnatural stimulus which activates in a synchronous fashion many types of peripheral nerve fibers responsive to innocuous as well as noxious stimuli; and 3) Animals learn to terminate and escape near-painful stimuli (Campbell and Masterson, 1969; Vierck et al, 1971).

With these problems in mind, we have developed a reaction time paradigm in monkey which has the following attributes. First, it utilizes positive and negative reinforcement and eliminates the tendency of animals to avoid rather than escape noxious stimuli. The animal is trained to detect the termination of an innocuous temperature increase (less than 45°C) in order to receive a reward on each trial. On trials in which the temperature increase reaches the noxious heat range (45° to 51°C), the monkey can escape the stimulus, but receive no reward. The monkey's operant response thus is dependent on stimulus intensity and motivational or drive state. Since the monkey initiates each trial, noxious stimuli cannot be avoided without eliminating opportunities for reward. Anticipatory responses also reduce rewards. Second, this paradigm provides two measures,

escape latency and escape probability, which can scale the
range of behavior to innocuous and noxious heat stimuli.
Third, it employs a natural stimulus, noxious heat, that is
more easily quantified than noxious mechanical stimuli.
Noxious heat also activates a more restricted group of peripheral and central neurons than mechanical stimuli (Dubner,
Sumino and Starkman, 1974).

    All of the above factors are critical for carrying out
one of our primary goals: the correlation of escape behavior with peripheral and central neuronal events in awake
monkeys. However, as we will show below, the monkey's escape performance also is sensitive to motivational shifts
independent of sensitivity to the sensory stimulus. This
animal model thus can be used to advantage in evaluating
the effect of various pharmacological and non-pharmacological analgesic agents on the sensory and reaction components
of the pain experience (Melzack and Casey, 1968).

                    BEHAVIORAL OBSERVATIONS

    The experimental situation is illustrated in Fig. 1.
A Rhesus monkey was placed in a restraining chair and its
head was fixed to the chair to reduce movements. A spring-
loaded contact thermode was applied to the upper lip region
and a liquid reward could be provided in calibrated increments through a metal tube placed in the mouth (Fig. 1,
upper left). The thermode contacted a 1-cm diameter, cir-
cular area of facial skin, and was precisely-controlled to
present temperature changes of 9°C/sec in the range of 20°
to 60°C. The thermode was located in the same general position for all trials.

    The monkey initiated a trial by depressing a trans-
lucent panel button after the light behind it was turned on
(Fig. 1, lower left). When the button was depressed, the
temperature at the surface of the thermode was increased at
a rate of 9°C/sec until it reached a predetermined final
temperature. The monkey received a grape juice reward if
the button was depressed until the return of the thermode
temperature to the baseline level. Figure 2 shows the sequence of events in greater detail. The arrows indicate
the start of the trial and the three possible behavioral
outcomes. Once the trial was initiated, the temperature

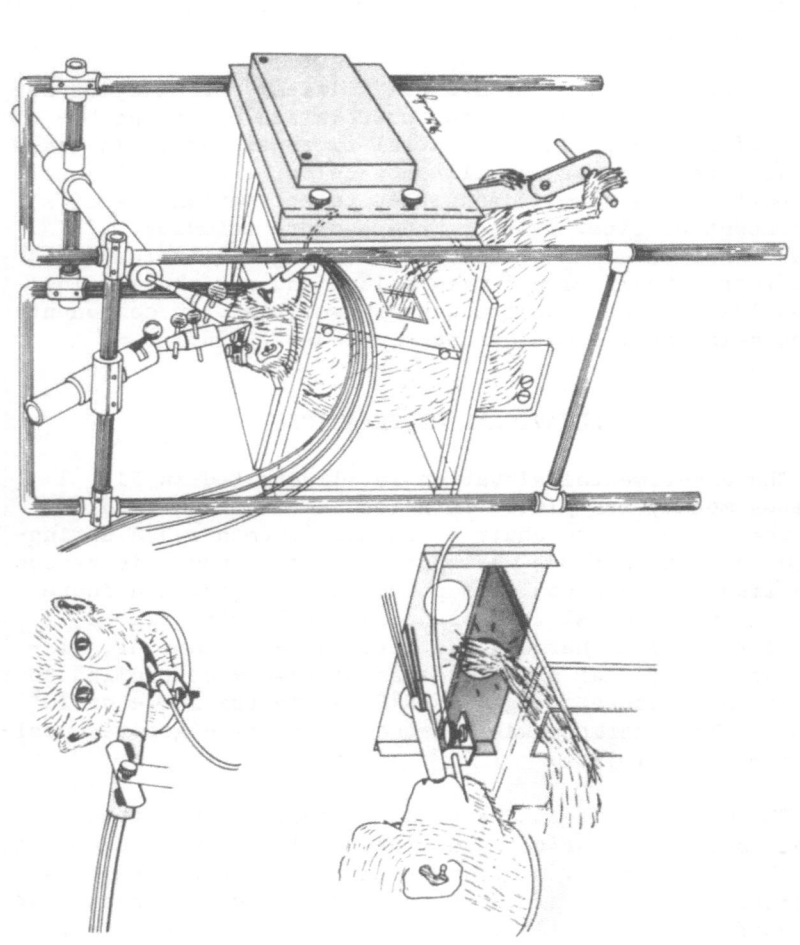

Fig. 1. Drawings of the experimental arrangement. See text for details.

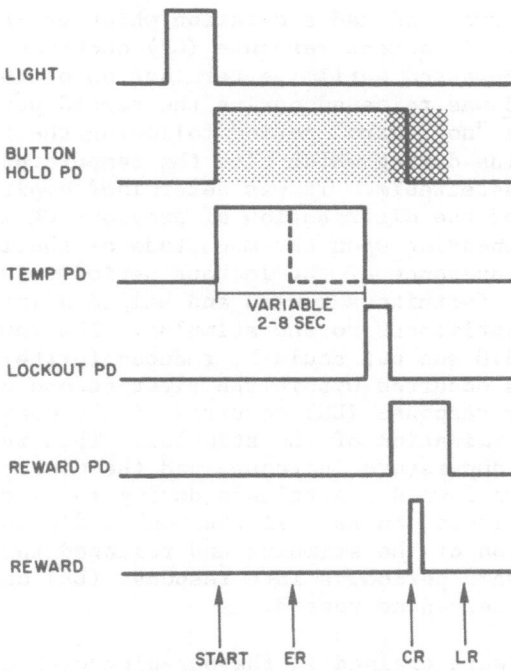

Fig. 2.   Sequence of events in the behavioral paradigm.   The
arrows indicate the start of the trial and the three possible behavioral outcomes: correct response (CR), early response (ER) and late response (LR).   The light behind the
panel button indicated to the monkey that a trial could be
started.   It turned off when the trial was initiated by the
monkey.   The "button hold pd" is the total period of time
the button was depressed.   The "temp pd" is the period or
duration of the temperature step which varied randomly from
2-8 sec.   The "lockout pd" was a period of 0.7 to 2.0 sec
after termination of the stimulus during which time the
temperature change was not detectable.   It increased in
duration with increases in the magnitude of the temperature
change.   The "reward pd" is the time period during which the
monkey had to release the button to receive a reward.   It
was 3.0 sec in duration.   The reward pulse activated a sole-
noid-controlled valve and provided the monkey with 0.3-0.5
cc of grape juice.   The minimum time between release of the
button and the start of the next trial was 15 sec.   See text
for further details.

increase occurred and had a duration which varied randomly
from 2-8 sec. A correct response (CR) occurred if the
button was depressed until the termination of the temperature step and was released during the reward period. The
lockout was a "no reward" period following the termination
of the stimulus during which time the temperature change
was not yet detectable. It was determined empirically from
an analysis of the distribution of previous CR latencies
and varied depending upon the magnitude of the temperature
change. The presence of the lockout period reduced the time
available for fortuitous reward and helped maintain the
monkey's attentiveness to the stimulus. The reward period
was kept at 3.0 sec but could be reduced further since almost all CR's occurred within the first second of the period. An early response (ER) occurred if the monkey released
before the termination of the stimulus. This release terminated the temperature increase, and the monkey received
no grape juice reward. A release during the lockout period
also was considered an ER. If the monkey did not detect
the termination of the stimulus and released the button
after the reward period, a late response (LR) occurred and
the monkey received no reward.

Monkeys were trained in the paradigm with a random
order of temperature increases of 2° to 11°C depending upon
the baseline or adapting temperature (30°, 35°, or 37°C).
Final temperatures never were greater than 43°C. After CR
probabilities of 95% or greater were achieved, temperature
increases into the noxious heat range (45° to 51°C) were
initiated on one-sixth of the trials. Noxious heat trials
were inserted quasi-randomly in the sequence of temperature
increases with the restriction that two such trials did not
occur consecutively. In addition, on noxious heat trials
the duration of the temperature period was fixed at 5 sec,
the mean duration of temperature steps for all trials.
This procedure eliminated variability in escape probabilities and latencies due to changes in the duration of the
noxious heat stimulus. On noxious heat trials, the monkey
had the choice of either escaping the stimulus by releasing
early (ER), and receiving no reward, or depressing the
button until the temperature increase terminated, and receiving a reward.

Figure 3 summarizes data collected from a Rhesus monkey who received water ad libitum in the home-cage and was

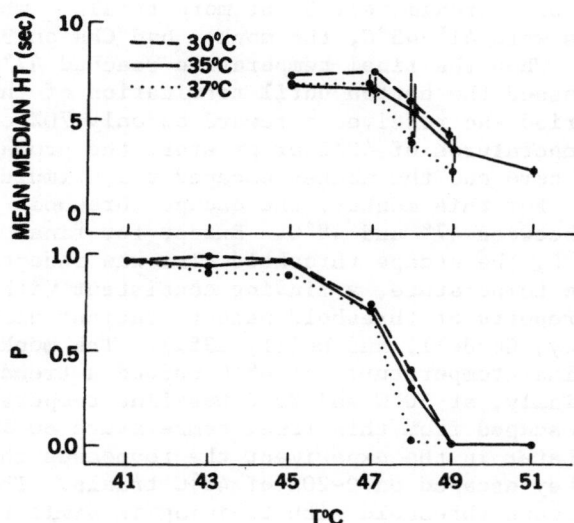

Fig. 3. Summary data from a Rhesus monkey that received water _ad libitum_ in the cage. The curves in both graphs represent data collected from three baseline temperatures: 30°, 35°, and 37°C. The upper curves show the hold times (total time the button was depressed) for temperatures of 41° to 51°C. Medians were determined from ten trials at each final temperature and mean median values (data points) and standard deviations of the median (extent of vertical lines) are shown. Means are based on at least 5 median values. The lower curves show the probabilities of CRs for final temperatures of 41° to 51°C. Each data point is based on approximately 50 or more trials.

rewarded with 0.3 cc of grape juice for each CR in the restraining chair. The lower graph shows the probabilities
of CRs (depressing the button until termination of the temperature period and releasing during the reward period) to
final temperatures of 41° through 51°C, from baseline temperatures of 30°, 35°, and 37°C. Each data point is based on
the outcome of approximately 50 or more trials. When final
temperatures were 41°-45°C, the monkey had CRs on 90-95% of
the trials. When the final temperature reached 47°C, the
monkey depressed the button until termination of the temperature period and received a reward on only 70% of trials.
By final temperatures of 49°C or greater, the probability
of a CR was zero and the monkey escaped the stimulus on all
the trials. For this monkey, the escape threshold (the 50%
level) was between 47° and 48°C. Except for final temperatures of 48°C, the escape threshold also was independent of
the baseline temperature, a finding consistent with human
subjective reports of threshold pain to radiant heat stimulation (Hardy, Goodell, and Wolff, 1951). The monkey's response to final temperatures of 48°C showed a trend over
time. Initially, at 30°C and 35°C baseline temperatures
the monkey escaped from this final temperature 80-100% of
the time. Later in the experiment the responses changed
and the monkey escaped on 0-20% of 48°C trials. This increase in escape threshold with training is similar to findings in human subjects who report higher pain thresholds
after gaining experience in the testing procedure (Neisser,
1959). However, there appears to be an increase in sensitivity at the 37°C adapting temperature. The monkey consis-
tently escaped this stimulus throughout the training procedure.

The curves in the upper graph of Fig. 3 also show the
tendency for increased sensitivity at higher baseline temperatures. They show the mean median hold times (HT; the
total time the button is depressed) and standard deviations
of the median for the 45° to 51°C final temperature trials.
Final temperatures above 47°C resulted in shorter HTs. HTs
also were inversely related to baseline temperature at final
temperatures of 48° and 49°C. This change in HT at 35° and
37°C baseline temperatures was greater than that predicted
from differences in time necessary to reach final temperatures. The mean median HTs in 49°C trials from 35° and
37°C baseline temperatures were 3.40 and 2.25 sec, respectively, whereas the time from baseline to final temperature

differs by 0.22 sec. It appears from these data that hold
time was dependent on baseline and final temperature and
provides another measure of escape behavior to varying intensities of noxious heat.

Another measure of escape behavior was provided by lip
movements during each trial. They were monitored by a sensitive accelerometer attached to the thermode. Figure 4
shows that lip movements associated with noxious heat
stimulation correlated with escape thresholds. The deflections in the upper trace of each record represent these
movements and those in the lower trace show the onset and
termination of each temperature step. Movements after the
termination of the temperature period resulted from lip
activity during consumption of the liquid reward. When
final temperatures were 48°C or greater, lip movements occurred before termination of the stimulus. These movements
probably represent a more reflexive motor act to escape the
stimulus than does release of the panel button. The data
indicate convergence of escape thresholds at 47° to 48°C
when assessed by these two measures.

The outcome was very different when the monkey's water
needs during the experimental period were changed. Figure
5 summarizes the data from another monkey under conditions
of water satiation and water restriction (200 cc per day).
In the satiated condition, the escape threshold was between
47° and 48°C from a baseline temperature of 35°C. Hold
times decreased at higher final temperatures. In the water-
restricted condition, however, the monkey depressed the
panel button until termination of the temperature period and
received a reward on 70-100% of trials irrespective of the
final temperature. Escape thresholds were higher than 51°C.
The actual escape threshold under the water-restricted condition was not determined because final temperatures above
51°C produce noticeable tissue irritation or damage.

Lip movements in the water-restricted condition continued to occur when final temperatures were 48°C or greater and were similar to lip movements in the water-satiated
condition (Fig. 6). Thus, the monkey's escape performance
is sensitive to changes in motivational or drive state.
However, sensitivity to the noxious stimulus appears unchanged when assessed by lip movements during the two conditions. The behavioral paradigm, therefore, provides a

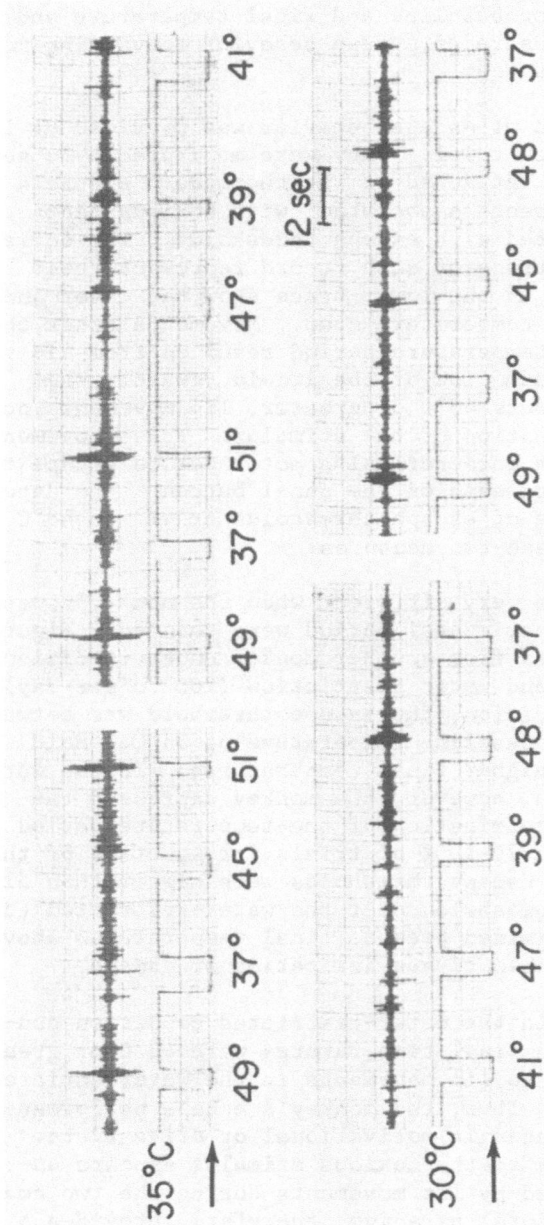

Fig. 4. Records of deflections produced by lip movements monitored by an accelerometer attached to the contact thermode. Upper trace in each record represents these movements and the lower trace indicates the onset and termination of each temperature period. Baseline temperature was 35°C in upper records and 30°C in lower records. Final temperature on each trial is indicated. Time calibration is 6 sec for each major division.

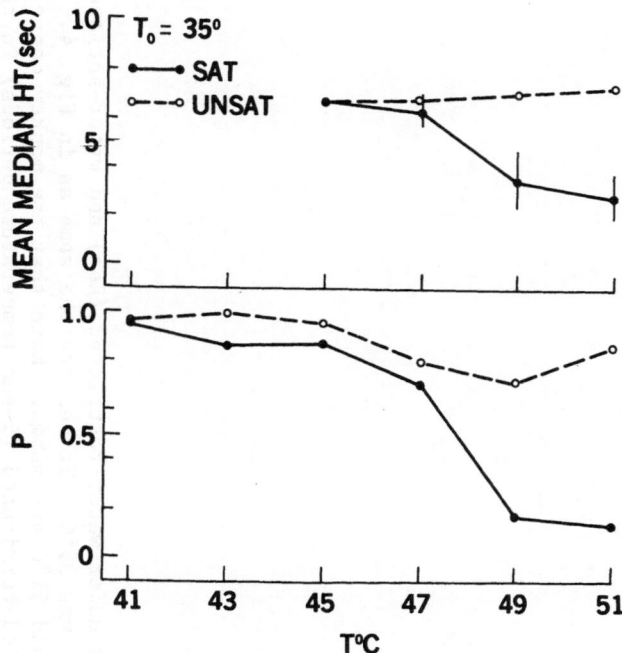

Fig. 5.   Summary data from a Rhesus monkey under conditions
of water satiation (SAT) and water restriction (UNSAT).
Baseline temperature was 35°C.   Ordinate and abcissa of each
graph are the same as in Fig. 3.   In the water-satiated condition, median values were determined from 4-5 trials each
and means from 5 median values.   In the water-restricted condition, median values were determined from 5-10 trials each
and means from three median values.   Each data point in the
probability curves is based on 20 or more trials.

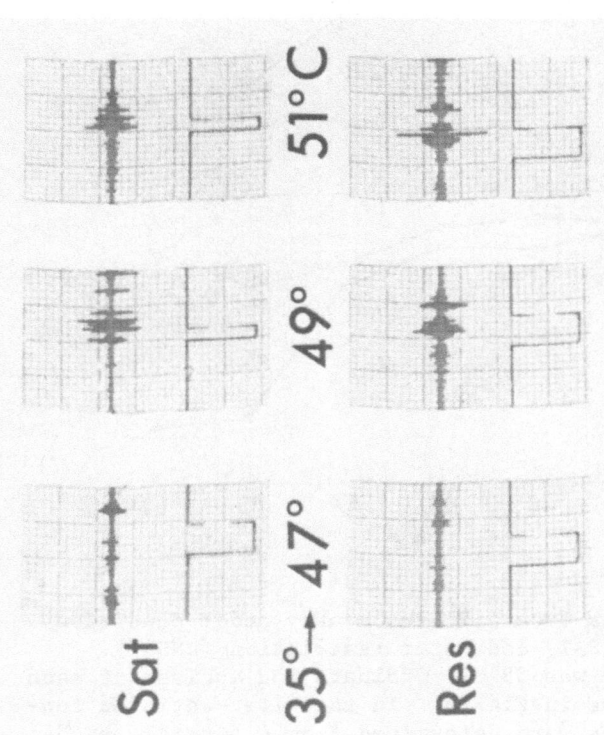

Fig. 6. Records of lip movements under water-restricted (Res) and water-satiated (Sat) conditions. Baseline temperature was 35°C. Traces are the same as in Fig. 4. Trials to final temperatures of 47°, 49°, and 51°C are shown. Note that the monkey depressed the button until the temperature period terminated (5-sec temperature periods) in the Res condition and received a reward on each trial. In the Sat condition, the monkey released the button early on the 49° and 51°C trials and did not receive a reward. Lip movements were similar in both Sat and Res conditions. Time calibration is 6 sec for each major division.

means of separating "pain sensitivity" from "pain response."
The effect of analgesic agents on these behavioral measures
in both of these drive conditions will be of considerable
interest. The differential responsiveness of neurons in
central "pain pathways" during the above manipulations also
warrants intense study.

Subjective reports of pain in humans to radiant heat
stimulation occur in the 44°-48°C range (Hardy, Jacobs, and
Meinner, 1953; McKenna, 1958; Neisser, 1959). We assessed
human subjective reports of pain utilizing the above behavioral paradigm and contact thermode. The subjects were
instructed to release the panel button whenever they felt
a pricking or burning pain. They were further instructed
not to tolerate or hold through any painful stimuli. Subjects were rewarded with the knowledge of correct responses
to thermal stimuli on each trial. The summary data from
three subjects is shown in Fig. 7. Reported pain thresholds
in 2 of 3 subjects were between 47° and 48°C and thus similar to that of the monkeys. Hold times decreased at higher
final temperatures. It appears that this behavioral paradigm produces escape and reflexive motor behavior in monkeys
over a range of noxious heat intensities similar to those
intensities at which humans report pain.

SUMMARY AND CONCLUSIONS

A behavioral animal model has been described for the
study of escape behavior in Rhesus monkey to noxious heat
stimuli. This escape behavior occurs over the range of
stimulus intensities at which humans subjectively report
pain under identical stimulus conditions. A number of other
measures, such as escape probabilities, escape latencies and
lip movements also converge to indicate that noxious heat
stimuli above 47°C are aversive to the monkeys. The model
has the following advantages: (1) It utilizes positive and
negative reinforcement and eliminates the tendency of animals
to avoid painful stimuli by escaping from nonpainful stimuli.
(2) The paradigm provides measures of escape behavior be-
sides escape probability which can be related to baseline
temperature and a range of noxious heat stimuli.   (3) A natural stimulus, noxious heat, is employed and data can be compared with psychophysical experiments of pain sensitivity
in humans to radiant heat (Hardy, Wolff, and Goodell, 1952).
(4) Escape thresholds are sensitive to motivational shifts

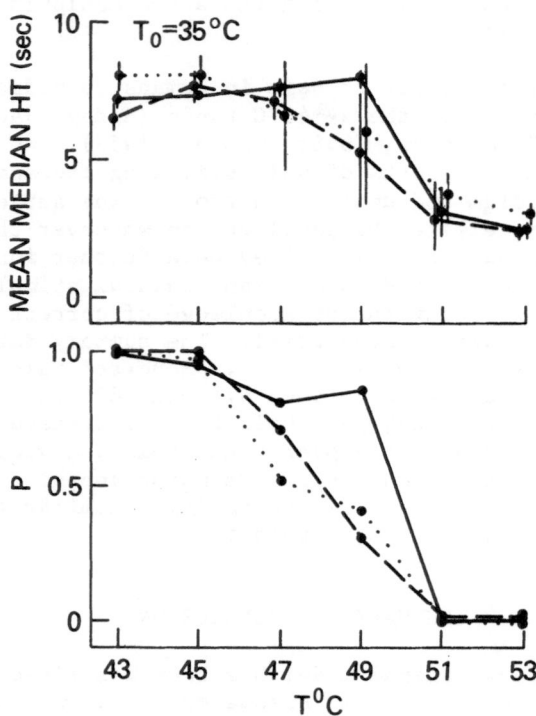

Fig. 7. Summary data from 3 human subjects instructed to
give subjective reports of pain in the same behavioral
paradigm and with the same contact thermode. Baseline temperature was 35°C. Ordinate and abcissa of each graph are
the same as in Fig. 3. Each curve represents the data from
a different subject. Median values were determined from
5 trials each and means from four or five median values.
Each data point in the lower graph is based on 20 or more
trials.

independent of any change in the monkey's sensitivity to the noxious heat stimulus.

The paradigm is now being used to correlate peripheral and central neural activity in the trigeminal system with the monkey's behavioral performance. The ability of the paradigm to separate sensitivity and reaction to noxious stimuli by motivational manipulation also should be useful in assessing the mechanisms of action of analgesic drugs and non-pharmacological methods of pain control.

REFERENCES

1. Burgess, P.R. and Perl, E.R.: Cutaneous mechanorecep-tors and nociceptors. In: Handbook of Sensory Phys-iology, Somatosensory System, edited by A. Iggo, Heidelberg: Springer-Verlag, 1973, 2:29-78.
2. Brown, A.G.: Effects of descending impulses on trans-mission through the spinocervical tract. J. Physiol., London, 1971, 219:103-125.
3. Campbell, B.A. and Church, R.M. (eds.): Punishment and Aversive Behavior, New York: Appleton-Century-Crofts, 1969.
4. Campbell, B.A. and Masterson, F.A.: Psychophysics of Punishment. In: Punishment and Aversive Behavior, edited by B.A. Campbell and R.M. Church, New York: Appleton-Century-Crofts, 1969, p. 3-42.
5. Casey, K.L., Keene, J.J., and Morrow, T.: Bulborecti-cular and medial thalamic unit activity in relation to aversive behavior and pain. In: Advances in Neurology, Pain, edited by John J. Bonica. New York: Raven, 1974, 4:197-205.
6. Dubner, R., Sumino, R., and Starkman, S.: Responses of facial cutaneous thermosensitive and mechanosensi-tive afferent fibers in the monkey to noxious heat stimulation. In: Advances in Neurology, Pain, edited by John J. Bonica. New York: Raven, 1974, 4:61-71.
7. Hardy, J.D., Goodell, H., and Wolff, H.G.: The influ-ence of skin temperature upon the pain threshold as evoked by thermal radiation. Science, 1951, 114: 149-150.

We are extremely grateful to Henry Burris, Mark Goddard, and Robin Harris for their excellent assistance in carrying out these experiments.

8. Hardy, J.D., Jacobs, I., and Meinner, M.D.: Thresholds of pain and reflex contraction as related to noxious stimulation. J. Appl. Physiol., 1953, 5:725-739.

9. Hardy, J.D., Wolff, H.G., and Goodell, H.: Pain Sensations and Reactions. Baltimore: Williams and Wilkins, 1952.

10. Manning, A.A. and Vierck, C.J., Jr.: Behavioral assessment of pain detection and tolerance in monkeys. J. Exp. Anal. Behav., 1973, 19:125-132.

11. McKenna, A.E.: The experimental approach to pain. J. Appl. Physiol., 1958, 13:449-456.

12. Melzack, R. and Casey, K.L.: Sensory, motivational and central control determinants of pain. In: The Skin Senses, edited by D.R. Kenshalo. Springfield: Thomas, 1968, p. 423-439.

13. Neisser, U.: Temperature thresholds for cutaneous pain. J. Appl. Physiol., 1959, 14:368-372.

14. Price, D.D. and Mayer, D.J.: Neurophysiological characterization of the anterolateral quadrant neurons subserving pain in M. Mulatta. Pain, 1975, 1:59-72.

15. Vierck, C.J. Jr., Hamilton, D.M., and Thornby, J.I.: Pain reactivity of monkeys after lesions to the dorsal and lateral columns of the spinal cord. Exp. Brain Res., 1971, 13:140-158.

16. Willis, W.D., Trevino, D.L., Coulter, J.D., and Maunz, R.A.: Responses of primate spinothalamic tract neurons to natural stimulation of hindlimb. J. Neurophysiol., 1974, 37:358-372.

17. Zimmermann, M. and Handwerker, H.O.: Total afferent inflow and dorsal horn activity upon radiant heat stimulation to the cat's footpad. In: Advances in Neurology, Pain, edited by John J. Bonica, New York, Raven, 1974, 4:29-33.

THE DEVELOPMENT OF A PAIN PERCEPTION PROFILE:

A PSYCHOPHYSICAL APPROACH

Bernard Tursky

New York State University at Stony Brook

Stony Brook, New York

Recently I visited the laboratory of a prominent neurologist who is involved in highly sophisticated nerve conduction research. He also maintains a private practice and is much sought after as a specialist and consultant. We talked about his research and he proudly described to me in great detail the complexities of his laboratory equipment, which had the appearance of a miniature space program launch facility. He was very articulate about his ability to manipulate all the physical and experimental variables in his research and took pains to explain how carefully he measured and controlled noise in his recording system. Our conversation finally shifted to my interests and I described some of my ideas about the need for developing methods to evaluate the individual patient's perception of pain. I asked him how he made such evaluations in his medical practice and what special instruments he used for this purpose. His answer was to reach into his pocket and solemnly produce a large safety pin which he identified, with almost the same amount of pride as he had expressed for his complex laboratory instruments, as his major test instrument in evaluating his patients' pain sensitivity. I do not have any objection to my friend's use of the safety pin but, if he is going to use it as a clinical test instrument, I, as a concerned scientist, want to know how the instrument is calibrated. That is, how sharp is the pin and how much force is used to prick the patient.

This little anecdote illustrates what must be regarded as a paradoxical situation. The medical and engineering

171

sciences, in recent years, have joined forces and spent a
great amount of effort and money in the development of research and diagnostic instruments to measure and record human vital functions. Physicians use these instruments in
their workups of patients to record various types of information pertinent to the individual's well-being. Accurate records are kept of each patient's height; weight;
acuity of vision, hearing, and reflexes; as well as the
patient's cardiovascular functions and blood chemistry.
These records are kept on a continuing basis and are used to
aid the physician in his diagnosis of pathological conditions.

It can, therefore, be regarded as strange that until
quite recently the verbal and behavioral expressions and
descriptions of pain, which clinicians rely on as proven
indicators of pathology, have been treated in almost cursory
fashion, and little has been done to develop scales and
instruments to scientifically evaluate and utilize these
important indicators of disease.

Recently there has been an increased interest in both
clinical and experimental approaches to the evaluation and
control of human pain. Several pain clinics have been organized to bring together medical, physiological, and psychological expertise to clinically investigate and attempt to
control intractable human pain and suffering. Symposia,
meetings, and workshops* have been organized to exchange

---

*International Symposium on Pain held at the University of
Washington School of Medicine, Seattle, Washington, May 21-
26, 1973. Proceedings of the symposium published as Volume 4 of the Advances in Neurology series, edited by Dr.
John Bonica, published by Raven Press, New York, 1974.
American Association for the Advancement of Science spon-
sored a symposium at the 1974 meetings in San Francisco and
the 1975 meetings in New York City. The 1974 proceedings
are to be published under the title The Control of Pain,
edited by M. Weisenberg, published by Psychological Dimensions, Inc., New York. Proceedings of the 1975 meeting to
be published under the title Pain: Therapeutic Approaches
and Frontiers of Research, edited by M. Weisenberg and B.
Tursky, published by Plenum Press, New York.

and disseminate information related to the understanding
and alleviation of human pain. This increased interest in
the study of pain has led to the organization of The International Association for the Study of Pain and the formation
of an international Pain journal for the publication of reviews and original research papers on the nature, mechanisms,
and treatment of pain. These activities have produced evidence of the clear need for a common language that can be
used by scientists, clinicians, and patients to communicate
information about the human pain experience. There is also
a need for the development of simple procedures that can be
used to define and quantify the individual patient's pattern
of pain responsivity. The methodology for obtaining this
information should be available to the clinician to enable
him, in a short examination period, to record for each individual patient a personal pain perception profile.

        Several attempts have been made recently to develop
such profiles. Shealy and Shealy (this volume), in their
chapter entitled "Behavioral Techniques in the Control of
Pain," report the use of a pain profile which attempts to
get at five areas of pain information, the percent of time
that pain is present, the severity of the pain, the effect
of pain on physical activity, the effect of pain on the use
of drugs, and the effect of pain upon the individual's mood.
Patients are asked to respond on a 5-point category scale
to indicate their position on each of these dimensions.
Fordyce (1976) is concerned with the behavioral analysis of
chronic pain. He suggests that a behavioral analysis of
each patient's pain problems is necessary and that psychological testing procedures be used to evaluate the various
factors that contribute to chronic pain. Fordyce proposes
the use of psychological evaluation procedures and the use
of a diary that records the individual's medication intake
and physical activity on an hourly and daily basis. Such
pain profiles are useful but they fail to provide information about the individual's pattern of pain responsivity.
One might argue that a pain perception profile should generate information related to how each individual judges and
reacts to a number of discrete pain perception variables.
These evaluation steps should provide information about the
patient's tactile threshold, his perception of several nociceptive levels of stimulation, his ability to psychophysically evaluate tactile stimulation ranging in intensity
from perception threshold to pain tolerance, and finally,

an evaluation of his ability to use language to meaningfully
describe his pain experience.

Progress has been made in the laboratory to develop
techniques for the study of human pain, and methodology already exists to accurately assess some of the pain profile
items suggested above. Specifically, a variety of controlled non-invasive laboratory stimulation procedures have
been developed: thermal (Hardy, Wolff & Goodell, 1952),
ischemic pressure (Smith, Lowenstein & Beecher, 1968), controlled pressure to a pressure sensitive area such as the
fingernail bed (Forgione & Barber, 1971), and electrical
stimulation combined with stabilized electrode-skin impedance (Tursky, 1974). Clark and Bindra (1956) determined
the pain threshold and tolerance levels of a group of subjects for electrical, thermal, and mechanical (pressure)
pain stimulation. They found large individual differences
between subjects for these pain measures under all three
stimulation modalities, but found strong within-subject
correlations across stimulation methods. The use of these
controlled stimulation techniques in conjunction with the
utilization of sophisticated psychophysical measurement
procedures makes it feasible to evaluate the quantitative
(intensity) component and qualitative (reactive) component
of the pain experience at various nociceptive levels.

Tursky, Greenblatt, and O'Connell (1970) utilized
electric shock and a method of limits scaling procedure to
accurately measure individual sensation thresholds. Other
studies (Sternback & Tursky, 1965; Higgins, Tursky & Schwartz,
1971; and Tursky, Greenblatt & O'Connell, 1970) indicated
that sensation thresholds for electrical stimulation are
extremely stable within individuals across time and locus of
stimulation, vary little between normal individuals, and are
not significantly affected by psychological factors. However, it has been demonstrated (Frankenhaeuser, Mellis &
Froeberg, 1967; Tursky, Greenblatt & O'Connell, 1970) that
strong electrical stimulation applied to the test site can
temporarily raise the tactile threshold level at that location. These findings are analogous to the auditory fatigue
found by Licklider (1951) since they both occur locally at
the peripheral level.

The evaluation of higher levels of noiception are more
complex than tactile thresholds. The qualitative and

quantitative elements of these measures interact to present
a difficult measurement problem. The techniques utilized
to measure the various designations of "pain" threshold have
been reviewed extensively (Beecher, 1959; Sternbach, 1968;
and others). Among these techniques is the work of Hardy,
Wolff, and Goodell (1952) who developed a scale to measure
the individual's pain perception thresholds for thermal
stimulation. They identified three levels of pain percep-
tion--pricking, burning, and aching pain--and found large
differences between individual judgments of these pain levels.

     Clark (1969) utilized signal detection theory developed
by Green and Swets (1966) to evaluate the separate contribu-
tions of the discriminative behavior of an individual's
sensitivity (d') and response criterion (Lx) in his pain
responses. Clark used signal detection to evaluate the
effect of a placebo described as a potent analgesic on both
the thermal sensitivity and subjective criterion for pain.
Clark and Mehl (1971) evaluated the effect of age and sex
on the d' of various pain response criteria. Clark and
Dillon (1973) used signal detection theory analyses to test
several types of pain judgments, and in a recent study Clark
and Yang (1974) used signal detection methods to evaluate
tolerance for thermal pain under acupuncture analgesia.
Their results indicated that the sole effect of acupuncture
is to raise the subject's criterion (Lx) for what is called
painful stimulation while the threshold for pain (d') is
not altered.

     A second psychophysical scaling procedure utilized to
evaluate the intensity of nociceptive laboratory stimulation is magnitude estimation. S. S. Stevens (1957) developed the magnitude estimation procedure to establish power
functions related to a number of perceptual continua such
as sound, light, and heat. In this procedure, the subject
is required to estimate the intensity of a series of equal
interval stimuli of a physical modality as they compare to
a standard stimulus in that modality. This procedure has
been utilized to evaluate the intensity of pain delivered
by both thermal and electrical stimulation. Stevens and
Stevens (1960) demonstrated that the relationship between
human estimates of the intensity of thermal stimulation
and the actual delivered temperature are adequately described by a series of power functions which are related
to the exposed skin area. Stevens and Marks (1971)

recently confirmed this finding and demonstrated that the
smaller the stimulated area, the greater the exponent of
the generated function. The exponent increases from 1.0
for a large stimulation area to 1.6 when the area is sub-
stantially decreased. Intensity and area interact to evoke
the same sensation of heat over much of the range.

Stevens, Carton, and Shickman (1958) investigated the
power function for electrical stimulation and reported a
power function with an exponent of 3.5. This function
seemed psychologically unsound since it seemed inconsistent
with the exponents of the functions of other skin stimulation modalities reported by Stevens (1961). For example,
vibration produces an exponent of 0.6 and warmth produces
an exponent of 1.6. Sternbach and Tursky (1964), using
Stevens' magnitude estimation technique with a fixed standard, reliably produced exponents from 1.6 to 1.94 depending
on the range of shock stimuli used. That is, judgments of
the intensity of shock stimuli grow in magnitude as the
increase in intensity of the stimulus raised approximately
to the 1.8 power. These findings seemed to be electrically
consistent since, with impedance anchored at 5000 ohms, the
delivered power increased as the square of the current.
The 1.8 exponent is close enough to the square function to
support the idea that, under these controlled conditions,
delivered power becomes the electrical parameter. That
probably controls the perceived intensity of the stimulus
as suggested by Hill, Flanary, Kornetsky, and Wikler (1952).

A recent study in the Laboratory for Behavioral Research
(Cross, Tursky & Lodge, 1975) utilized numerical magnitude
estimation, force of handgrip, and sound pressure as response measures to estimate the intensity of a random series
of electric shocks. The validated exponent of the function
generated in the study was approximately 2.2, again close
to the function generated by Sternbach and Tursky (1964)
and further supporting the theory that perceived intensity
is related to delivered power. This lawful metric relationship between stimulus intensity and magnitude estimation
has been demonstrated to be consistent across various subject populations such as college students (Sternbach &
Tursky, 1964) and groups of housewives (Sternbach & Tursky,
1965), thus providing a psychophysical method for evaluating
individual and group expressions of the intensity of pain.

Other procedures have been utilized to evaluate the intensity of clinical pain. Sternbach, Murphy, Timmermans, Greenhoot, and Akeson (1974) recently developed a subjective pain estimate procedure with which pain patients estimate the severity of their usual clinical pain on a scale of 0 to 100. This pain estimate is then compared with a ratio computed from the subjects' exposure to the submaximum effort tourniquet technique (Smith, et al., 1968). The tourniquet pain ratio is computed by having the patient match the intensity of the induced ischemic pain to that of his usual clinical pain and then continue until the ischemic pain becomes intolerable. Sternbach's data indicate that the ischemic pain measures are highly reliable in normal, low-back pain patients and a series of patients with mixed chronic pain symptoms, but that the pain estimate is reliable only in the chronic pain group. The pain estimate produced by this procedure is greatly decreased by surgical treatment for pain relief and only slightly reduced by psychological treatment. The tourniquet ratio decreases with surgical treatment but increases with psychological treatment, seeming to reflect actual pain perception.

Although these psychophysical measurement procedures have been useful in evaluating the intensity of laboratory stimulation and, in some instances, clinical pain, we are still faced with the problem of interpreting and quantifying the most common mode of communication related to information about the pain experience--the individual's use of language to describe the various aspects of his pain experience. Perhaps the greatest problem that confronts the pain researcher is the development of instruments to evaluate information that is provided in the form of verbal self-report.

The language used to describe pain is varied and useful. For example, the use of burning as opposed to aching as a sensory pain descriptor may convey to the clinician information indicating whether the pain felt by the patient is related to a nerve injury or to a more visceral complaint. Despite the universal use of verbal report to describe pain, very little has been done to categorize or evaluate the intensity of pain-descriptive words.

In our laboratory, the terms discomfort, pain, and tolerance have been utilized in several studies (Nichols &

Tursky, 1967; Higgins, et al., 1971) as indicators for de-
finable levels of pain perception. These verbal indicators
of nociceptive levels were tested for reliability in two
well-controlled studies. In one study (Tursky & O'Connell,
1972), subjects were required to identify their discomfort,
pain, and tolerance levels as the electrical stimulus intensity delivered to each of three concentric electrodes
was raised in small steps. Several determinations were
made on each electrode in two separate experimental sessions.
The range of intensities for each suprathreshold level across
subjects was extremely wide. For example, pain tolerance
levels varied from as low as 2.4 ma to as high as 14.0 ma.
However, highly significant Pearson product-moment correlations ranging from 0.89 to 0.99 were derived from each
suprathreshold measure between runs on the same day. Similar comparisons between corresponding runs between days
produced slightly lower, but still highly significant,
correlations at all suprathreshold levels of intensity. The
high degree of reliability produced by these pain connota-
tive judgments indicates that the individual psychic reaction to pain is stable from day to day, and, therefore, it
should be possible to reliably evaluate each individual's
judgment of pain levels.

     In a second study (Price & Tursky, 1975), the effect
of varying the duration and increment of increase of electrical stimulation on the reliability of these subjective
nociceptive judgments was tested. The findings of the previous study related to the reliability of discomfort, pain,
and tolerance judgments were confirmed. Although the success of these efforts is gratifying, it is possible that
words like discomfort and pain are generic in their assessment of nociception. That is, these words may not distinguish between intensity and reaction. Therefore, it would
be useful to develop word scales that can be used to independently assess the magnitude of each of these pain-
descriptive categories.

     Melzack and Torgerson (1971) and Melzack (1976), made
an effort to separate the use of pain-descriptive terms
into three pain categories. One hundred and two terms relating to pain were obtained from the clinical literature and
separated into three major categories as follows:

     (1) words describing the sensory qualities of the
          pain experience--pricking, burning, or stinging;

(2) words describing the affective qualities of the
     pain experience in terms of tension, fear, or
     autonomic properties--sore, tender, or splitting;
     and

(3) evaluative words describing the subjective,
     overall intensity of the pain--annoying,
     discomforting, or excruciating.

Groups of doctors, patients, and students were asked
to assess these terms on a 7-point category scale of intensity. A high level of agreement was demonstrated among the
judges on the relative intensity of each term. Melzack and
Torgerson's efforts constituted a major step in the evaluation of pain descriptors; however, it would have been of
even greater value if such pain evaluative responses had
been psychophysically scaled and their relative magnitudes
clearly established.

Recently, the Laboratory for Behavioral Research in
the Political Science Department at the State University of
New York at Stony Brook has been conducting a research program devoted to the development of cross-modally validated
psychophysically sound verbal scales for evaluating the
perceived importance of political and social phenomena
(Lodge, Cross, Tursky & Tanenhaus, 1975). In this effort,
magnitude estimation procedures were utilized to evaluate
sets of adjectives that have been used in Likert-type
category scales to describe the importance and support for
political or social events, institutions, and decisions.

Magnitude estimation has been defined as the simplest,
most direct, and currently the most widely used method of
constructing scales with ratio properties. Subjects are
presented with a series of test stimuli, one at a time in
random order, and are required to render numerical judgments proportional to the magnitude of the sensations evoked
by each stimulus. Analysis of the data developed from many
experiments discloses a consistent pattern: magnitude of
sensation grows as a function of some power of stimulus intensity. This does not imply that all modalities produce
the same power function. In fact, in most instances, exponents vary rather widely. For example, the exponent of
numerical estimates of line length is 1.0; for force of
handgrip, 1.7; and for sound pressure, 0.67. What the

psychophysical power law implies is a simple lawful relationship between stimulus intensity and sensory response:
equal stimulus ratios should produce equal subjective ratios.

The use of numbers as a response measure raises some
questions about the validity of the power law. Stevens and
his associates developed a validation procedure known as
cross-modality matching (Stevens & Mach, 1959). This procedure calls upon the subject to match the apparent magnitude of a response in one physical modality (e.g., force of
handgrip) to the intensity of a stimulus in another modality
(e.g., the loudness of sound). As the investigator alters
the intensity of sound pressure, the subject squeezed the hand
dynamometer to match the apparent alteration in loudness.
When the subjective value of a range of responses in one
modality is set equal to the subjective value of a range of
stimuli in another modality, the exponent for the power
function described by this relationship should be equal to
the ratio between the established exponents of the two
modalities. Since the exponent for loudness established by
numerical magnitude estimation is 0.67 and the exponent for
handgrip is 1.7, the matched data should produce a new
power function of 0.39. This validation procedure has been
confirmed for many physical stimuli.

Magnitude estimation procedures have been utilized to
scale many physical stimulus modalities, but more impor-
tantly, in recent years investigators have utilized the
same procedures to scale many dimensions of social consensus
(Stevens, 1975). Dawson & Brinker (1971) employed a cross-
modality (handgrip and sound pressure) matching technique
to validate magnitude estimation scales of the degree of
racism in a number of racial statements. When handgrip
matches were plotted against loudness matches, the resulting relationship was well-approximated by a power function
equal to 0.39, the predicted ratio of the handgrip and loudness exponents.

Of course, the verification of a known psychophysical
relationship by an indirectly established cross-modality
matching relation is not evidence that the separate psychophysical scales are valid measures of psychological magnitude, as, for instance, the degree of racism expressed by
each of the statements used in the Dawson and Brinker experiment. It must be further demonstrated that the empirical

scales constructed from the loudness and handgrip matches
are both free of <u>regression</u> bias. This bias is a tendency
for a person's judgments to regress toward a mean level,
thus underestimating large magnitudes and overestimating
small ones (Stevens & Greenbaum, 1966). The typical effect
of this bias is to produce power functions with lower exponents. It has been shown that this bias occurs as a
power transformation on the matching variable and, under a
certain set of circumstances, its effects can be calculated
and removed from the data (Cross, 1974).

It was decided to utilize the cross-modality matching
procedures to develop and evaluate three sets of pain descriptors that could be used to describe the intensity,
reactive, and sensory aspects of the human pain experience.
The intensity scale was defined as a measure of <u>how much the
pain hurts</u> in units of intensity, the reactive scale was
defined as a measure of <u>how unpleasant the pain feels</u> in
units of reaction, and the sensory scale was defined as a
measure of <u>what the pain feels like</u> in units of sensation.
The selection of descriptors for each scale was based on a
series of pretests: the first served to sort a large number of descriptors, including many used by Melzack and
Torgerson (1971), into three categories, and subsequent
tests used simple, verbal magnitude estimation procedures
in large classrooms to evaluate each scale. The results of
the classroom scaling procedure were used to eliminate descriptors that demonstrated too much variability in classi-
fication or estimation. These pretests provided a number
of words in each descriptor category that offered the best
range in the three classes of descriptors. The intensity
descriptors ranged from <u>just noticeable</u> to <u>excruciating</u>,
the reactive descriptors ranged from <u>bearable</u> to <u>agonizing</u>,
and the sensation descriptors ranged from <u>tingling</u> to <u>pierc-
ing</u>.

The three sets of pain descriptors were embedded in
simple sentences, each beginning with <u>The pain is</u>, and a
full-scale study was conducted to construct a cross-modally
validated, bias-free scale for each of the three categories
of pain descriptors. The procedure used to evaluate these
descriptors is similar to that used by Lodge, et al. (1975)
and Cross, et al. (1975).

Fifty-six undergraduate students took part in this

study. The stimuli presented to the subjects were three
sets of slides shown on a rear-projection screen placed in
front of the subject. Each subject was seated in a comfortable lounge chair. Mounted on the arm of the chair was a
sone potentiometer which controlled the amplitude of noise
delivered to a set of earphones worn by the subject. The
maximum level of deliverable noise was set at 100 db. An
electrical analog of the sound pressure was recorded on one
channel of a Beckman dynograph to provide a permanent record
of each response. Also mounted on the arm of the chair was
a 100-kg. handgrip dynamometer. This instrument was designed to test and record the subject's handgrip responses.
Built into this device was a potentiometer which turned in
conjunction with the handgrip spring, thus providing an
electrical output proportional to the tension on the spring
of the dynamometer. This response was also recorded on the
dynograph. Located in front of the subject under the rear-
projection screen were three illuminable boxes labeled Talk,
Squeeze, and Noise. The box that indicated the expected
response was illuminated two seconds before the slide came
on. Subjects were presented with three sets of stimuli.
The first was a set of six log interval line lengths. The
responses to these physical stimuli provided information
for correcting the regression bias of the functions generated by the non-metric pain descriptors.

Each subject was presented with the full range of lines
and then with two of the three sets of pain descriptors.
The combination of stimulus sets and the order of presentation within each set were randomized across all subjects.
Judgments of apparent line length and magnitude of intensity,
reaction, and sensation were estimated separately using the
three response measures: magnitude estimation, handgrip,
and sound pressure. In each modality, the subject produced
a response proportional to the magnitude of each stimulus
relative to a standard. Number estimates were given verbal-
ly, sound level was adjusted by the subject using the sone
potentiometer, and the dynamometer was used to produce
squeeze responses. A fourth response was added at the end
of the experiment when each subject was asked to draw lines
proportional to the same pain descriptor statements. Finally, each subject was required to judge the same two sets
of pain descriptors on standard 9-point category scales.
These procedures provided five response measures related
to the proportional intensity of each stimulus.

The results of this study were found to be consistent and significant, and the information for the calibration data and each descriptor category is reported in some detail.

Calibration. The geometric means of the magnitude estimation, handgrip, and sound pressure responses to the six line lengths were calculated. The expected theoretical exponents of each of the functions for each subject group are 0.67 for sound pressure, 1.0 for magnitude estimation, and 1.7 for handgrip. The actual exponents of the generated functions averaged across all groups were 0.68 for sound pressure, 1.03 for magnitude estimation, and 2.01 for handgrip. The differences between the theoretical and obtained exponents can be interpreted as indicators of regression bias and can be used to correct for this bias in evaluating the pain descriptor scales.* The product-moment correlations

---

* Its seems clear from the standpoint of our expectations concerning these psychophysical relations that, in the construction of a scale based on the obtained psychophysical response measures, allowance must be made for regression effects. Failure to take regression bias into account results in an attenuation or compression of estimated scale values, a nonlinear displacement of the theoretically true values toward an average level. The biased scale values were computed as the geometric means of the three psychophysical scale values assigned to each stimulus item which, in turn were derived from the ME, SP, and HG response measures by raising each to its theoretically correct exponent (1.0, 0.67, and 1.7). Expressed as an equation:

$$\psi = K(ME^{1.0}SP^{0.67}HG^{1.7})^{1/3}$$

where K is a scale constant selected so the standard stimulus is assigned the arbitrary modulus of 50 units of support. These scale values are considered to be biased to the extent that, because of psychophysical regression, the component response measures either underestimate or overestimate the true strength of support expressed by an item. The true scale values were computed in the same manner with an important difference in the exponents in the equation: empirically derived multiplicative parameters correcting the regression bias were computed from the line length data and used to transform the exponents for each psychophysical scale as in the follow equation:

$$\psi = K(ME^{a(1.0)}SP^{b(0.67)}HG^{c(1.7)})^{1/3}$$

between pairs of response measures for all groups range
from 0.98 to 0.998.

Pain Descriptors. Figure 1 shows a plot of the functions generated for the words in the intensity scale. In
this instance, since words do not have a known metric responses cannot be plotted directly against words. Instead,
the calculated scale values were utilized as a surrogate metric. These derived scales have a theoretical exponent of
1.0, thus the geometric means of the magnitude estimation,
handgrip, and sound pressure responses should produce approximately their expected theoretical functions when plotted
against these scale values.

The product-moment correlations between response modes
for the fifteen stimuli are extremely high: magnitude estimation to handgrip, 0.989; magnitude estimation to sound
pressure, 0.994; and handgrip to sound pressure, 0.980. The
exponents and ratios of the sound pressure, handgrip, and
magnitude estimation functions fall within the 95 percent
confidence limits of the expected functions.

The responses to the reactive and sensory descriptors
produced similar results. All product-moment correlations
between response measures ranged from 0.960 to 0.990 and the
exponents of all response functions for both scales fell
within the 95 percent confidence limits.

The geometric means of line production responses drawn
by each subject at the end of the session were computed
across subjects for each stimulus and plotted against the
geometric means of the magnitude estimation responses for
the same stimuli. Theoretically, the predicted relationship between these functions should be unity. The slopes
of the regression lines for log magnitude estimation and
log line production are 1.11 for the intensity scale, 1.08
for the reaction scale, and 1.3 for the sensory scale. The
product-moment correlations for these measures range from
0.993 to 0.997. This is an important finding because line
production and numerical magnitude estimation are relatively
simple psychophysical response measures that can easily be
utilized in the field or clinician's office to calibrate
individual pain descriptor responses.

A question that must be raised is, "Why go to all this

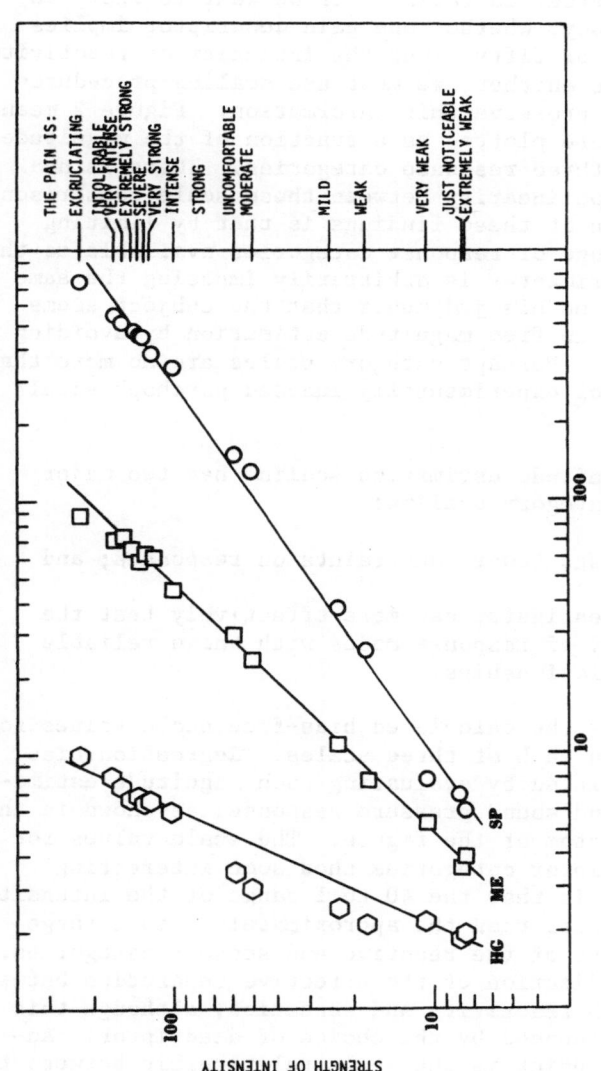

Figure 1. Strength of Intensity v. Relative Magnitude of Response. Handgrip (HG), Magnitude Estimation (ME), and Sound Pressure (SP) responses (x-axis) as a function of the strength of intensity of pain (y-axis) based on all three response measures, each corrected for regression. Each point is the geometric mean of twenty responses.

trouble? Why not simply evaluate these descriptors by use
of simple category scales?" The answer is that category
scales, rating scales, or partition scales cannot answer
questions about perceived ratios. If we want to know, as
in the present study, whether one pain descriptor implies
twice, ten times, or fifty times the intensity or reactivity
for pain than does another, we must use scaling procedures
that draw out and preserve this information. Figure 2 mean
category ratings are plotted as a function of the magnitude
data for each of three response categories. There is no
question of the nonlinearity between these scale comparisons.
One interpretation of these findings is that by limiting
the number and range of response categories available to the
subject, the experimenter is arbitrarily imposing the same
kind of restraint on his judgments that the subject seems
to impose himself in free magnitude estimation by avoiding
extreme responses. Perhaps category scales are no more than
extreme examples of experimentally induced psychophysical
regression.

Clearly, magnitude estimation scaling has two major
advantages over category scaling:

(1) It imposes fewer constraints on responses; and

(2) The investigator can more effectively test the
     validity of response modes with known reliable
     interrelationships.

Table 1 shows the calculated bias-free scale values for
the descriptors in each of three scales. Regression bias
correction is achieved by evaluating each magnitude estimation, handgrip, and sound pressure response, as shown in the
formula at the bottom of the figure. The scale values for
each of the descriptor categories show some interesting
differences. One is that the 40 to 1 range of the intensity
scale is much greater than the approximately 7 to 1 range
of the scale values of the reactive and sensory categories.
This may be an indication of the effective separation between
intensity and both reactivity and sensation, although this
effect may be influenced by the choice of descriptor. Another interesting point is the scale relationship between the
descriptors _uncomfortable_ and _intolerable_ which, as I pointed
out, had been used in several previous studies as descriptors
of reactivity to pain. In this instance, these words were

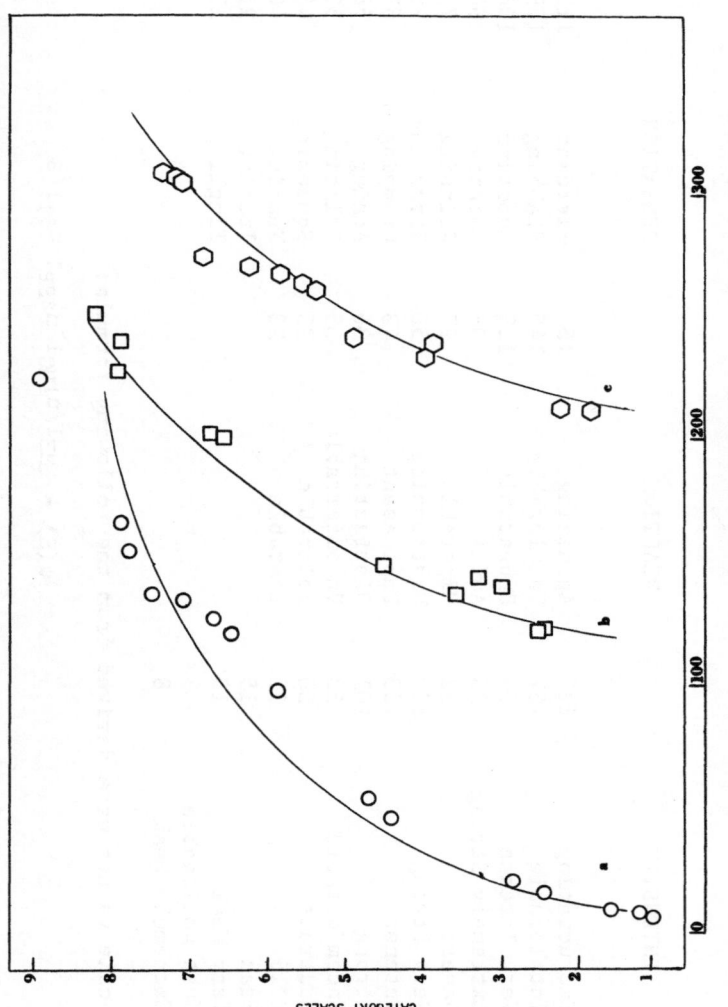

Figure 2. Category v. Magnitude Scales of (a) Intensity, (b) Reaction, and (c) Sensation. The curves represent the best fitting logarithmic functions. Magnitude scales have been displaced by 100, 200, or 300 units for clarity.

TABLE 1

RELATIVE SCALE VALUES FOR THREE DIMENSIONS OF PAIN

INTENSITY		REACTION		SENSATION	
*Excruciating	227	Agonizing	153	Piercing	113
Intolerable	167	Intolerable	145	Stabbing	109
Very Intense	154	Unbearable	128	Shooting	106
Extremely Strong	135	Awful	98	Burning	80
*Severe	132	Miserable	97	Grinding	79
Very Strong	129	Distressing	50	Throbbing	75
Intense	123	Unpleasant	43	Cramping	67
*Strong	101	Distracting	36	Aching	58
Uncomfortable	58	Uncomfortable	35	Stinging	50
*Moderate	50	Tolerable	23	Squeezing	46
*Mild	23	Bearable	23	Numbing	40
*Weak	15			Itching	25
Very Weak	10			Tingling	17
*Just Noticeable	8				
Extremely Weak	8				

*Scale values were derived from the following formula:

$$\psi(S) = (ME^{1/n_1}HG^{1/n_2}SP^{1/n_3})^{1/3}$$

embedded in both the intensity and reactive descriptor scales. Despite the fact that the two scales were judged by different groups of subjects, the scale distance between the two words is almost identical for both categories, although the ratio between them is greater in the reaction scale than in the intensity scale. These results demonstrate that our assumption of the generic pain descriptor qualities of these words is reasonable.

This chapter presents an idea that may be of importance to both the clinician and the patient. The development of a set of evaluation steps to define and quantify each individual's pattern of pain responsivity might make it possible for the physician to prescribe and treat conditions that produce pain and suffering more effectively. The steps suggested in this chapter are reasonable and well within the framework of our present abilities for implementation. As stated in the beginning, the profile steps should provide information about the patient's stimulation threshold, his perception of several nociceptive levels of stimulation, his ability to psychophysically evaluate tactile stimulation ranging from threshold to pain tolerance levels, and his ability to use language to meaningfully describe his pain experience. The following procedure might be followed to achieve these goals:

1. The patient receives a standard physical examination to determine that he is not suffering from some physical or neural impairment that might be aggravated by the administration of the pain perception profile.

2. Test for Sensation Threshold--an accurate measure of the individual's threshold for laboratory stimulation. The patient is required to psychophysically identify the level of stimulation at which he first perceives any sensation. This test provides a basis for determining the normality of the individual's neural transmission pathways. The use of controlled and quantifiable low-level tactile stimulation (electrical, thermal, or pressure) and an appropriate psychophysical scaling technique (method of limits, signal detection) applied to both sides of the body would establish the sensitivity and bilateral symmetry of the patient's perception of tactile stimulation.

3. Determination of Individual Nociceptive Stimulation

Levels--an accurate measure of the amount of controlled
stimulation that each patient rates as being <u>uncomfortable</u>,
<u>painful</u>, and the level at which he voluntarily refuses to
<u>tolerate</u> any further increase in stimulation. Stimulation
is increased in small steps until each nociceptive level is
reached. Instructions stressing the voluntary nature of
these determinations must be included and each pain measure
should be determined twice to insure a true assessment.

4. Determination of the Patient's Ability to Psychophysically Judge the Intensity of Tactile Stimulation.
Five log interval stimulation steps based on the difference
between the individual's threshold and tolerance stimulation
levels can be presented to the patient for evaluation using
a magnitude estimation procedure. The median stimulus can
be designated as a standard and arbitrarily assigned a
standard response value in each response modality. The patient would then be required to judge each of the five levels
of stimulation aginst the standard in each response mode.
The five stimuli can be rapidly presented three times in
random order for each response mode. The geometric means
of the three judgments in each response mode can be averaged
and individual, cross-modally validated power functions can
be calculated. This procedure should provide information
related to the individual's ability to make stable judgments
about the intensity of painful stimulation.

5. The Psychophysical Evaluation and the Use of a
Standard Set of Pain Descriptors Related to the Intensity,
Reactivity, and Sensory Components of the Pain Experience.
Using a technique similar to that used to evaluate the
nociceptive stimulation levels, each patient would be required to psychophysically judge a subset of the descriptors
listed in Table 1. He would then be asked to assign an intensity descriptor to each of the levels of stimulation
used in step 4 of the profile. Other sets of terms related
to unpleasantness and sensory evaluation of the stimuli
could also be provided to form a word diagram of the patient's
assessment of each stimulation level.

The tools to obtain the information related to the individual pain perception profiles are, for the most part,
now available. A major effort must still be made to develop
and test any missing components and to demonstrate in the
laboratory the feasibility of this approach to the assessment

of individual pain perception. It is not suggested, however, that these proposed evaluation items are the only or
best parameters to be utilized in producing an individual
pain profile.

Instead, I propose that these steps be considered as a
point of reference for other investigators. Much additional
research must be conducted before we can determine whether
the suggested steps will produce the best measures for build-
ing individual pain profiles. The population utilized for
most of the described studies is made up of normal college
students; further research must be conducted using younger,
older, and clinical populations to establish the effect of
these variables on the suggested pain reactions. We are
presently working with a group of chronic migraine headache
sufferers both in the laboratory and at home. Studies are
being conducted on the consistency of their pain responses.

It is hoped that this report will trigger an interest
by other pain researchers to replicate and extend our research findings. It is only through such an exchange of
ideas and information that we can evolve the best methods
to evaluate and alleviate human pain and suffering.

REFERENCES

Beecher, H.K. Measurement of subjective responses: quanti-
    tative effects of drugs. New York: Oxford University
    Press, 1959.
Clark, J.W. & Bindra, D. Individual differences in pain
    threshold. Canadian Journal of Psychology, 1956, 10,
    69-76.
Clark, W.C. Sensory-decision theory analysis of the placebo
    effect on the criterion pain and thermal sensitivity
    (d'). Journal of Abnormal Psychology, 1969, 74, 363-371.

This effort was supported by National Institute of Mental
Health Grant #MH-22296-04 and National Science Foundation
Grant #S041125. The author wishes to thank the staff of
the Labroatory for Behavioral Research at the University of
New York at Stony Brook for their able assistance.

Clark, W.C. & Dillon, D.J.   SDT analysis of binary decisions
and sensory intensity ratings to noxious thermal stimuli.
Perception and Psychophysics, 1973, 13, 491–493.

Clark, W.C. & Mehl, L. Thermal pain: a sensory decision
theory analysis of the effect of age and sex on d', various response criteria, and 50% pain threshold. Journal
of Abnormal Psychology, 1971, 78, 202–212.

Clark, W.C. & Yang, J.C. Acupunctural analgesia? Evaluation by signal detection theory. Science, 1974, 184,
1096–1098.

Cross, D.V. Some technical notes on psychophysical scaling.
In H. Moskowitz, B. Scharf & J. C. Stevens (Eds.), Sensation and measurement: paper in honor of S. S. Stevens.
Dordrecht, Holland: D. Reidel Publishing Co., 1974,
23–26.

Cross, D.V., Tursky, B. & Lodge, M. The role of regression
and range effects in determination of the power function
for electric shock. Perception and Psychophysics, 1975,
18, 9–14.

Dawson, W.E. & Brinker, R.P. Validation of ratio scales
of opinion by multimodality matching. Perception and
Psychophysics, 1971, 9, 413–417.

Fordyce, W.E. Behavioral methods for chronic pain and illness. Saint Louis: C. V. Mosby Co., 1976.

Forgione, A.G. & Barber, T.X. A strain gauge pain stimulator. Psychophysiology, 1971, 8, 102–106.

Frankenhaeuser, M., Mellis, I. & Froeberg, J. Effect of
electrical stimulation on sensation threshold. Perceptual and Motors Skills, 1967, 24, 271–275.

Green, D.M. & Swets, J.A. Signal detection theory and psychophysics. New York: John Wiley & Son, 1966.

Hardy, D.J., Wolff, H.G., & Goodell, H. Pain sensations
and reactions. Baltimore: Williams and Wilkins, 1952.

Higgins, J.D., Tursky, B. & Schwartz, G.E. Shock elicited
pain and its reduction by concurrent tactile stimulation.
Science, 1971, 172, 866–867.

Hill, H.E., Flanary, H.G., Kornetsky, C.H. & Wikler, A. Relationship of electrically induced pain to the amperage
and the wattage of shock stimuli. Journal of Clinical
Investigation, 1952, 31, 261–266.

Licklider, J.D.R. Basic correlates of the auditory stimulus.
In S. S. Stevens (Ed.), Handbook of Experimental psychology. New York: John Wiley & Son, 1951, 985–1039.

Lodge, M., Cross, D., Tursky, B. & Tanenhaus, J. The psychophysical scaling and validation of a political support scale. American Journal of Political Science, 1975, 19, 611–649.

Melzack, R. The McGill Pain Questionnaire: major properties and scoring methods. Pain, 1, 277–299.

Melzack, R. & Torgerson, W.S. On the language of pain. Anesthesiology, 1971, 34, 50–59.

Nichols, D.C. & Tursky, B. Body image, anxiety, and tolerance for experimental pain. Psychosomatic Medicine, 1967, 29, 103–110.

Price, K.P. & Tursky, B. The effect of varying stimulus parameters on judgments of nociceptive electrical stimulation. Psychophysiology, 1975, 12, 663–666.

Smith, G.M., Lowenstein, D. & Beecher, H.K. Experimental pain produced by the submaximum effort tourniquet technique: Further evidence of validity. Journal of Pharmacology and Experimental Therapeutics, 1968, 163, 468–474.

Sternbach, R.A. Pain: a psychophysiological analysis. New York: Academic Press, 1968.

Sternbach, R.A., Murphy, R.W., Timmermans, G., Greenhoot, J.H. & Akeson, W. Measuring the severity of clinical pain. Advances in Neurology, 1974, 4, 281–288.

Sternbach, R.A. & Tursky, B. On the psychophysical power function in electric shock. Psychonomic Science, 1964, 1, 217–218.

Sternbach, R.A. & Tursky, B. Ethnic differences among housewives in psychophysical skin potential responses to electric shock. Psychophysiology, 1965, 1, 241–246.

Stevens, J.C. & Mack, J.D. Scales of apparent force. Journal of Experimental Psychology, 1959, 58, 405–413.

Stevens, J.C. & Marks, L.E. Spatial summation and the dynamics of warmth sensation. Perception and Psychophysics, 1971, 9, 391.

Stevens, J.C. & Stevens, S.S. Warmth and cold: dynamics of sensory intensity. Journal of Experimental Psychology, 1960, 60, 183.

Stevens, S.S. On the psychophysical law. Psychological Review, 1957, 64, 153–181.

Stevens, S.S. To honor Fechner and repeal his law. Science, 1961, 133, 80–86.

Stevens, S.S. Psychophysics: introduction to its perceptual, neural, and social prospects. New York: John Wiley & Son, 1975.

Stevens, S.S., Carton, A.S. & Shickman, G.M. A scale of
    apparent intensity of electric shock. Journal of Experi-
    mental Psychology, 1958, 56, 328-334.
Stevens, S.S. & Greenbaum, H.B. Regression effect in psy-
    chophysical judgment. Perception and Psychophysics, 1966,
    1, 439-446.
Tursky, B. Physical, physiological, and psychological fac-
    tors that affect pain reaction to electric shock. Psy-
    chophysiology, 1974, 11, 95-112.
Tursky, B., Greenblatt, D.J. & O'Connell, D. Electrocutan-
    eous threshold changes produced by electric shock. Psy-
    chophysiology, 1971, 7, 490-498.
Tursky, B. & O'Connell, D. Reliability and interjudgment
    predictability of subjective judgments of electrocutan-
    eous stimulation. Psychophysiology, 1972, 9, 290-295.

PAIN SENSITIVITY AND THE REPORT OF PAIN: AN INTRODUCTION TO SENSORY DECISION THEORY

W. Crawford Clark

New York State Psychiatric Institute and
Columbia University
New York, New York 10032

The purpose of this paper is to introduce a new psycho-physical procedure for the objective measurement of experimental pain. This technique, known as "signal detection theory," or more descriptively, "sensory decision theory," distinguishes between a person's report of pain and his sensory experiences induced by noxious stimuli. Obviously, a procedure which permits the separation of the attitudinal component of the pain response from the sensory component should prove to be of great value to investigators studying the action of analgesics, and to physicians concerned with the problem of evaluating clinical pain. Sensory decision theory has recently been used to study the effects of placebos[1] and analgesics,[2,3] as well as sex and age[4] on experimental pain in man. However, a complete description of the theory and a detailed exposition of the calculations required to evaluate the variables defined by the mathematical model are not readily available. This paper provides an introduction to sensory decision theory by presenting in detail a segment of a larger study by Clark, Goodman, and Mehl[5] on the effects of suggestion on the pain

From anesthesiology 40:272-287, Copyright 1974. Reprinted by permission.

Supported in part by the National Institutes of Health through Grant NS09263 from the National Institute of Neurological Diseases and Stroke, and Grant RR05650 from the General Research Support Branch, Division of Research Facilities and Resources.

response to noxious thermal stimulation.

    Sensory decision theory emphasizes the distinction be-
tween the pain experience itself and an individual's criterion for reporting pain. An individual with a minor afflic-
tion who complains violently of pain sets a low criterion
for reporting pain, whereas a stoic has a high response criterion. The practitioner is constantly confronted with the
problem of evaluating the patient's report of pain. He must
distinguish between the psychological or attitudinal factors
which influence the response and the somatic component. For
it is well known that, in addition to being an objective
report of an internal state, a patient's report of pain may
be an expression of fear, a cry for help, a demand for attention, or an attempt to exert control over others. Anxiety, which according to Corman et al.[6] is present in a very
large proportion of patients undergoing operations, obviously plays an important role in increasing the complaint of
pain. If the physician reduces the patient's anxiety by
providing reassurance as recommended by Egbert et al.,[7] the
patient may be expected to report less pain and discomfort;
whether he experiences less pain is, however, a separate
issue. It is of paramount importance to recognize that the
report of pain is not the sensation of pain, for the report
is heavily influenced by the decision processes of the individual. The same amount of experienced pain may be described as painful in one instance, for example, if the patient is demanding the physician's sympathy and attention,
but not on another occasion, when the patient is attempting
to deny the presence of a serious illness.

    In contrast to clinical pain, where the intensity of
the pain stimulus is difficult to evaluate, experimental
pain lends itself to the study of the influence of psychological variables on the report of pain. In the study of
experimental pain the intensity of the physical stimulus is
determined with great precision, and the subject's responses
to the noxious stimuli are typically expressed as the pain
threshold. The pain threshold is the stimulus intensity at
which the subject reports the pain sensation to be present
with 50 percent of the stimuli. If the proportion of pain
reports is high, indicating great sensitivity to pain, the
subject is said to possess a low threshold to noxious stimulation. Conversely, few reports of pain indicate insensitivity and a high pain threshold. Experimental pain commonly

is thought to be altered by psychic factors, that is, cognitive control. For example, pain thresholds have been raised by placebos,[1] by redirection of the focus of attention,[8] by counterirritant auditory stimulation,[9] and by hypnosis.[10] The usual conclusion is that these raised thresholds reflect reductions in experienced pain. However, as sensory decision theory[11] has recently made clear, the traditional threshold is an extremely unreliable measure. The threshold is not a pure indicator of sensory sensitivity, because it is also influenced by the observer's response bias, that is, his eagerness or reluctance to report the presence of a stimulus independently of sensory experience. Clark[1,12] has hypothesized that many of the dramatic elevations in pain threshold reported in the literature reflect a response bias which lowers the proportion of pain responses rather than a change in the pain experience itself.

Sensory decision theory has been successfully applied to a wide variety of sensory problems,[13] as well as to problems of diagnosis in medical decision making.[14] The most important contribution of the theory is the division of the traditional threshold into two components. One component, d', provides a relatively pure measure of sensory discriminability which remains unaltered when variables such as attitude, expectation, and motivation are manipulated. A low d' means that the subject tends to confuse lower and higher intensity stimuli. A low d' results when the physical intensities of the stimuli are close together or when the subject's sensory system is insensitive. Thus, a decrease in d' following the administration of an analgesic suggests that the drug has actually attenuated neural activity in the sensory system(s). This interpretation is supported by the study of Chapman, Murphy, and Butler,[2] who recently showed that a mixture of 33 percent nitrous oxide with oxygen, when administered for a duration (15 min) sufficient to produce an analgesic effect, decreased d' in a group of volunteers exposed to noxious thermal stimulation. Dillon[3] obtained a similar result following the administration of aspirin.

The second measure of the subject's performance is the criterion which estimates the subject's response bias, or attitude. A high value indicates that he refuses to report his sensory experience as painful until he is quite certain that he is actually experiencing pain. From the viewpoint

of sensory decision theory, a subject with a high criterion
who has the same d' as a subject with a low criterion en-
dures the same amount of pain, but does not label it as
painful.

In an early application of sensory decision theory to
problems in pain perception, Clark[1] found that the administration of a placebo described as a potent analgesic sharply
decreased the proportion of pain responses to radiant-heat
stimulation, that is, the threshold for pain was raised.
However, analysis of the data by sensory decision theory
demonstrated that thermal discriminability, d', had remained
unchanged, and that the sole effect of the placebo was to
alter the subjects' criterion for reporting pain. Thus, the
reduced number of pain responses actually reflected an increase in the amount of noxious stimulation the subjects
were willing to endure before calling it pain, and not a
decrease in their sensitivity to noxious thermal stimuli.
This experiment demonstrated that it is imperative to use
sensory decision theory if meaningful conclusions concerning the relative influence of sensory sensitivity and response bias on the pain threshold are to be drawn. Previous
studies[8,9,10] in which nonsensory variables such as suggestion, attention, hypnosis, counterirritant stimulation, etc.
were found to influence the pain threshold clearly must be
re-examined, since sensory decision theory makes it manifest
that an altered pain threshold does not, as is usually in-
ferred, prove that pain sensitivity has been affected. It
is equally likely that such threshold changes merely reflect
an altered criterion for reporting pain. These considerations led to the design of the experiment reported below.

The present experiment was designed to investigate the
effects of suggestion, one form of cognitive control, on
thermal discriminability (d') and on the response criterion,
and to compare these results with changes in the traditional
threshold in the same subjects. The withdrawal response
was studied in addition to verbal report, since there is
some evidence that the withdrawal to a high-intensity stimulus more closely resembles the response to clinical pain
than does the report of just-perceived pain to a lower-intensity stimulus.

METHOD

Apparatus

Radiant-heat stimuli were presented by a Hardy-Wolff-
Goodell Dolorimeter (Williamson Development Co.) which had
been completely modified except for the gun-like projector,
housing a 100-watt projector bulb. The bulb was powered by
a programmable DC precision power supply which was accurate,
over an input range of AC 105 to 135 volts, to less than
0.15 percent or 1.0 millivolt (whichever is greater) for
load variations from 0 to 120 volts (Lambda Electronics
Corp. Model LH 131 FM). The duration of the stimulus was
3.00 sec. To measure withdrawal latencies a microswitch,
which was affixed to the tip of the projector housing,
stopped the clock and the stimulus if a withdrawal occurred
before 3.00 sec. The clock used a 600-Hertz fork-oscillator
with digital division to provide an accuracy of $\pm$ .01 sec.
The output of the lamp was calibrated daily, at each of the
stimulus intensities used, by means of a standard thermopile
(Williamson Development Co. Model RT2) and a potentiometer-
type galvanometer. The 2.0-cm diameter heat stimuli were
presented to six 3.0-cm patches of India ink applied to the
middle of the volar surface of each of the subject's fore-
arms. The subject moved the projector sequentially to each
patch as instructed by the experimenter. Six stimulus intensities were used: 0, 120, 240, 305, 370, and 435 mcal$\cdot$
sec$^{-1}\cdot$cm^{-2}. The stimuli were presented to a new patch every
15 sec to allow ample time (3 min) for the stimulated patch
to return to its initial temperature before being stimulated
again. Under these conditions, the skin temperatures measured at the beginning and end of each test period by a
thermistor (Yellow Springs Instrument Co. Model 43TD) were
31.0 and 31.2 C. Room temperature was maintained between
23 and 35 C.

Each subject served in a single session which was split
into an Initial Period (no attitudinal bias) and a Post-
suggestion Period (biased attitude) of 20 min each. During
each period 72 stimuli, 12 at each of six intensities, were
presented in a partially random ascending series of inten-

sities. The stimulus intensities were not completely randomized, since there is considerable evidence[15] that the
"anticipation of pain" induced by the progressively
increasing intensity increments characteristic of the method
of limits makes a significant contribution to the results
obtained, perhaps because anxiety is systematically increased.

Instructions

The subjects were ten paid college students. The instructions for the pre-suggestion period were minimal. The
subjects were informed that they were members of a non-drug
comparison group in a study of the analgesic effects of two
drugs. The following instructions were then given:

"We wish to determine your ability to feel warmth, heat,
and faint pain. A variety of heat intensities, including
zero, will be applied to your arm. Some stimuli will be so
weak that you will feel nothing at all, others will be hot,
while others will produce a painful sensation. If you feel
that the stimulus is getting too hot, remove the projector
from the skin. (Withdrawal times were recorded to the nearest .01 second.) Here is a list of possible responses to
help you maintain consistency." (See displayed material
below.)

The post-suggestion period followed a rest interval of
5 min. These instructions were designed to raise the criterion for pain tolerance, that is, to decrease the number
and speed of withdrawals:

"Our previous research indicates that repeated thermal
stimulation alters the ability to tolerate pain. Since the
previous thermal stimulation has fatigued your skin receptors
and made them less sensitive, you will now probably be more

Rating Scale for Categorizing Strength of Thermal Experience

Nothing	Detect	Faintly	Warm	Hot	Very	Very	Faint	Painful	Very	Withdrawal*
	Something	Warm			Hot	Faint	Pain		Painful	
						Pain				

* The Withdrawal category was used for analysis, but was not on the list presented to the subject.

able to endure the painful stimuli and withdraw the projector less frequently. Under the set of conditions in which
you are being tested, we are particularly interested in how
much pain you can tolerate before you must remove the projector. It is important for the purpose of the drug study
that we determine the maximum stimulation that you can endure. This is, then, a test of your ability to endure max-
imal pain."

     Two pain thresholds and response criteria were studied.
The verbal report of "very faint pain" locates the pain detection threshold, or the criterion for reporting a just
noticeable amount of pain. The withdrawal response defines
the pain tolerance threshold of the withdrawal criterion;
it measures the maximum amount of pain the subject is willing to endure. In the present study the instructions were
directed towards modifying only the criterion for withdrawal. Thus, changes in the withdrawal response are directly influenced by the instructions (Manipulated Response),
while changes in the verbal report of pain are not (Incidental Response).

                          RESULTS

     In this section, the data will first be examined from
the viewpoint of traditional psychophysical procedures.
Sensory decision theory will then be introduced, and the
computational procedures explained; finally, the results of
the experiment itself will be considered.

                 Traditional Threshold Analysis

     Table 1 shows the mean number of responses (averaged
over all subjects) made to each stimulus intensity before
and after the suggestion that more pain could be tolerated.
(The original data obtained from a typical single subject
closely resemble the stimulus-response matrix presented in
this table. For a single subject, the number of responses
in each cell divided by 12, the number of stimuli presented
at each intensity, yields the conditional probability that
a particular response will follow the occurrence of a particular stimulus.) The mean conditional probabilities,
averaged over all subjects, appear in Table 2. In general,

Table 1. Stimulus–Response Matrix: Mean Number of Responses, Averaged over All Subjects in Each Response Category to Each Stimulus Intensity before and after the Suggestion That More Pain Could Be Tolerated (Fewer Withdrawals)

						Response*					
	Nothing	D	FW	W	H	VH	VFP	FP	P	VP	Withdrawal
Stimulus intensity (mcal·sec⁻¹·cm²)											
Pre-suggestion											
435					.24	1.32		.24	1.56	1.20	9.00
370							.60	1.08	2.40	1.32	5.04
305		.12	.12	1.32	4.44	2.28	.60	.96	.60	.96	
240	.24	1.20	.48	3.00	4.80	.60	.36	.72	.36		.24
120	.84	2.04	4.92	3.48	.72						
0	7.44	3.12	.96	.24			.12				.12
Post-suggestion											
435					.24	.60	.24	.72	2.64	1.20	6.36
370				.12	1.56	1.92	1.68	1.20	1.92	1.68	1.92
305			.24	1.92	4.92	1.80	.36	.36	1.56	.60	.24
240	.24	.36	2.64	1.68	4.44	.12	1.44	.60	.24	.12	.12
120	1.20	2.76	5.64	.84	.60	.24	.60		.12		
0	6.96	4.32	.36	.12		.12	.12				

* The response categories are from the subject's Response Scale: D-Detect Something, F-Faint, W-Warm, H-Hot, V-Very, P-Pain.

Table 2. Stimulus–Response Matrix: Mean Conditional Probability of a Particular Response, Averaged over All Subjects, to Various Stimulus Intensities before and after the Suggestion That More Pain Could Be Tolerated

						Response*					
	Nothing	D	FW	W	H	VH	VFP	FP	P	VP	Withdrawal
Stimulus intensity (mcal·sec⁻¹·cm⁻²)											
Pre-suggestion											
435								.02	.13	.10	.75
370					.02	.11	.05	.09	.20	.11	.42
305		.01	.01	.11	.37	.19	.05	.08	.05	.05	.08
240	.02	.10	.04	.25	.40	.05	.03	.06	.03		.02
120	.07	.17	.41	.29	.06						
0	.62	.26	.08	.02			.01				.01
Post-suggestion											
435					.02	.05	.02	.06	.22	.10	.53
370				.01	.13	.16	.14	.10	.16	.14	.16
305			.02	.16	.41	.15	.03	.03	.13	.05	.02
240	.02	.03	.22	.14	.37	.01	.12	.05	.02	.01	.01
120	.10	.23	.47	.07	.05	.02	.05		.01		
0	.59	.36	.03	.01		.01	.01				

* The response categories are from the subject's Response Scale: D-Detect Something, F-Faint, W-Warm, H-Hot, V-Very, P-Pain.

the higher the stimulus intensity, the greater the probability of a pain response. Considerable imprecision, predicted by the theory and essential for data analysis, is present. Stimuli of the same physical intensity elicit a variety of responses: low-intensity stimuli are occasionally called painful and noxious stimuli are occasionally termed not painful. Also, stimuli of different intensities frequently receive the same response. For example, in the post-suggestion period the response Very Hot was applied to all stimulus intensities including zero.

A comparison of pre- and post-suggestion periods reveals that the suggestion that more pain could be tolerated before withdrawal produced the expected effect on the threshold for Withdrawal. The probability of a withdrawal to the 435 mcal·sec^{-1}·cm^{-2} stimulus decreased from .75 to .53 (matched $\underline{t}$=3.20, $\underline{df}$=9, $\underline{P}$ < .025) and the probability of a withdrawal to the 370 mcal·sec^{-1}·cm^{-2} stimulus decreased from .42 to .16 mcal·sec^{-1}·cm^{-2} (matched $\underline{t}$=3.27, $\underline{df}$=9, $\underline{P}$ < .01). For the pre- and post-suggestion periods, the withdrawal thresholds (50 per cent threshold, method of constant stimuli) are approximately 385 and 430 mcal·sec^{-1}·cm^{-2}, respectively. Thus, instructions which suggested that fewer withdrawals would be made because less pain would be felt (Manipulated Effect) significantly raised the withdrawal threshold by 45 mcal·sec^{-1}·cm^{-2}.

Table 3 presents the conditional probability data of table 2 successively cumulated from right to left. This procedure groups all responses indicative of pain detection (from Very Faint Pain to Withdrawal) from subjectively less intense sensory experiences (Nothing to Very Hot). A comparison of the pre- and post-suggestion periods reveals that the suggestion that more pain could be tolerated before withdrawal produced a minor effect on the threshold for the verbal report of pain (Incidental Threshold). The probability of a pain detection response to the 370 mcal· sec^{-1}·cm^{-2} stimulus decreased from .87 to .70 (matched $\underline{t}$ = 2.21, $\underline{df}$ = 9, $\underline{P}$ < .025) and the probability of a pain detection response to the 305 mcal·sec^{-1}·cm^{-2} stimulus decreased from .31 to .26 (matched $\underline{t}$ = .79, $\underline{df}$ = 9, $\underline{P}$ < .4). For the pre- and post-suggestion periods, the 50 percent thresholds for the verbal report of pain (see table 3) are approximately 330 and 340 mcal·sec^{-1}·cm^{-2}, respectively. Since the difference between responses at 305

Table 3.   Stimulus-Response Matrix: Mean Cumulated Conditional Probability of Responses to the Right of a Particular Category, Averaged over All Subjects, before and after the Suggestion That More Pain Could Be Tolerated

	Response*										
	Nothing	D	FW	W	H	VH	VFP	FP	P	VP	Withdrawal
Stimulus intensity $(\text{mcal} \cdot \text{sec}^{-1} \cdot \text{cm}^{-2})$											
Pre-suggestion											
435								1.0	.98	.85	.75
370					1.0	.98	.87	.82	.73	.53	.42
305		1.0	.99	.98	.87	.50	.31	.26	.18	.13	.08
240	1.0	.98	.88	.84	.59	.19	.14	.11	.05	.02	.02
120	1.0	.93	.76	.35	.06						
0	1.0	.38	.12	.04	.02	.02	.02	.01	.01	.01	.01
Post-suggestion											
435					1.0	.98	.93	.91	.85	.63	.53
370				1.0	.99	.86	.70	.56	.46	.30	.16
305			1.0	.98	.82	.41	.26	.23	.20	.07	.02
240	1.0	.98	.95	.73	.59	.22	.21	.09	.04	.02	.01
120	1.0	.90	.67	.26	.13	.08	.06	.01	.01		
0	1.0	.42	.06	.03	.02	.02	.01				

* The response categories are from the subject's Response Scale: D-Detect Something, F-Faint, W-Warm, H-Hot, V-Very, P-Pain.

$\text{mcal} \cdot \text{sec}^{-1} \cdot \text{cm}^{-2}$ failed to reach statistical significance, it is unlikely that the instructions, which were with respect to the withdrawal response, not the verbal report, exerted any influence on the verbal pain report threshold.

It is clear from tables 1, 2 and 3 that withdrawal responses were most frequent at 435 and 370 $\text{mcal} \cdot \text{sec}^{-1} \cdot \text{cm}^{-2}$, while cumulated pain detection responses predominated at 370 and 305 $\text{mcal} \cdot \text{sec}^{-1} \cdot \text{cm}^{-2}$. Only at these intensities did every subject respond with both pain detection and withdrawal responses, a prerequisite for statistical evaluation of the data. For this reason, these particular responses and stimulus intensities were selected from the entire stimulus-response matrix for detailed examination. In summary, the experiment demonstrated that suggestion raised the threshold for withdrawal to a painful stimulus. The question remains, however, whether this finding demonstrates that the instructions caused the subjects to actually experience less pain--the standard interpretation of a raised threshold--or whether the subjects experienced the same amount of pain but raised their criterion for withdrawal--a

possible alternative interpretation according to sensory
decision theory.

The next two sections provide a qualitative, and then
a quantitative, introduction to sensory decision theory.
Readers who do not wish to study the methodologic details
should proceed to the final section.

An Introduction to Sensory Decision Theory

The purpose of this section is to describe the rudi-
ments of sensory decision theory and to provide examples of
the calculations necessary to compute a value for sensory
discriminability (d'), and for the response criterion.
Additional details and a more detailed mathematical exposition appear elsewhere.[11,16,17] Sensory decision theory was
developed by communication engineers in order to describe
mathematically the performance of a "receiver" when the
task of the receiver is to distinguish between a time period
(observation interval) which contains a signal (with noise)
from one which contains no signal, that is, noise alone.
The term noise refers to interference or "static" which
resembles the signal. The source of this noise may be internal, for example, neural noise, or external, for example,
a sensory input of low intensity. Although this terminology
is confusing when applied to pain perception, it is firmly
established and will be adhered to here. In pain perception,
a higher-intensity stimulus is, on the average, relatively
more noxious than a lower-intensity stimulus, and is equivalent to a signal. Similarly, a lower-intensity stimulus
may be regarded as relatively innocuous, and is equivalent
to a blank. In this instance, activity in the fibers which
mediate the perception of warmth may be regarded as adding
neural noise to the pain system. With respect to responses:
"high," "pain," and withdrawal are equivalent to "yes"; and
"low," "not painful," and no withdrawal are equivalent to
"no" in a binary decision task. This stimulus-response
matrix appears in table 4. A positive response ("yes,"
"high," "pain," or withdrawal to signal-plus-noise (signal,
higher-intensity stimulus, or noxious stimulus) constitutes
a hit, while a positive response to noise alone (blank,
lower-intensity stimulus, or innocuous stimulus) yields a
false alarm. Misses and correct rejections are simply the
complements of hits and false alarms, and add no further
information.

Table 4.   Stimulus–Response Matrix
for Binary Decisions

	Responses	
	"No," or "Low," "No Pain," No Withdrawal	"Yes," or "High," "Pain," Withdrawal
High-intensity stimulus, I_2 (signal plus noise)	Miss	Hit
Lower-intensity stimulus, I_1 (noise alone)	Correct rejection	False alarm

　　　　Table 5 presents the cumulated conditional probabilities
of the responses of a single subject, from which values of
d' and the criterion are computed. In the pre-suggestion
period, the conditional probability of a withdrawal response
to the 435 mcal·sec^{-1}·cm^{-2} stimulus (hit probability) was
.80, and the conditional probability of a withdrawal response
to the 370 mcal·sec^{-1}·cm^{-2} stimulus (false-alarm probability)
was .36. A graphic example of this subject's performance,
as interpreted by sensory decision theory, is portrayed in
figure 1. The theory assumes that background interference,
termed "noise," is always present in amounts which vary
randomly overtime. This random process is assumed to be
represented by the unit normal probability density function,
or "normal distribution." Thus, when a moderate stimulus
of 370 mcal·sec^{-1}·cm^{-2} is presented, one of a broad spectrum
of subjective intensities, ranging from warm to painful, is
reported. This is portrayed graphically in the left-hand
("noise") probability density function in figure 1. The
abscissa represents the various intensities of subjective
experience, and the ordinate represents their probability
of occurrence. The observation or decision axis may be
viewed in a variety of ways: as frequency of neural impulses, as intensity of sensory experience, or as values of
the response criterion. In figure 1 the decision axis is
interpreted as intensity of sensory experience, that is, the
decision axis is the response scale: Nothing to Withdrawal.
When the higher-intensity stimulus of 435 mcal·sec^{-1}·cm^{-2}

is presented, the right-hand ("signal-plus-noise") density
function, with a higher mean, and with sensations ranging
from hot to extremely painful, is generated. The ordinate
represents the probability of occurrence of a particular
sensory experience along the abscissa. Thus, the magnitude
of each sensory experience along the observation axis (abscissa) has two probabilities associated with it, a probability that value arose from the lower intensity, or noise,
distribution and a probability that it arose from the higher
intensity, or signal-plus-noise, distribution. The subject's
problem is to decide whether a particular sensory experience
was more likely to have been caused by the lower-intensity
stimulus, or was more likely to have been caused by the
higher-intensity stimulus. Because these two distributions
overlap, the subject has no means of knowing in an absolute
way whether a given observation along the x-axis arose from
a low- or a high-intensity stimulus, and he must make a
statistical decision. (Thus, sensory decision theory views
the subject as a decision-maker confronted with a statistical choice based on probabilities; this position is in marked contrast to the traditional view that the subject "auto-
matically" responds when his sensory threshold is reached.)
Sensory decision theory postulates that in order to make his
decisions in a consistent manner, the subject chooses a cut-
off point, or response criterion. In the present example,
C_w represents the criterion for withdrawal from the stimulus. If the subject withdraws to the higher-intensity
stimulus he scores a hit, if he withdraws to the lower-
intensity stimulus he obtains a false alarm. Note that the
criterion splits the decision axis: all responses to the
right are Withdrawals and all responses to the left are No
Withdrawals, that is, the various verbal reports, "very
painful," "painful," "very hot," are grouped into a single
category. In figure 1 the probability of a hit appears as
the area (80 percent) under the high-intensity stimulus distribution to the right of C_w, and the probability of a false
alarm appears as the area (36 percent) under the low-intensity stimulus distribution to the right of the same criterion. The probability of a miss (20 percent) and the probability of a correct rejection (64 percent) form the areas
to the left of the criterion under the high- and low-intensity distributions, respectively. The hit and false-affirmative rates are sufficient to determine the two indices of
the subject's performance: his ability to discriminate between the two stimuli ($\underline{d}'$ = 1.20), and the locus of his

subjective criterion ($\underline{C}_w$ = 389.4). The procedures for calculating these measures are described in the next section.

The Mathematics of Sensory Decision Theory

In this section, graphic examples and mathematical definitions of the sensory decision theory indices are given, followed by specific examples from the data presented in table 5 and figure 1.

The manner in which $\underline{d}'$ varies as a function of hit and false-affirmative probabilities is portrayed in figure 2.

Table 5. Stimulus-Response Matrix for a Typical Subject: Cumulated Conditional Probability of All Responses to the Right of a Particular Category before and after the Suggestion That More Pain Could be Tolerated

	Response*										
	Nothing	D	FW	W	H	VH	VFP	FP	P	VP	Withdrawal
Stimulus intensity (mcal· sec⁻¹· cm⁻²)											
Pre-suggestion											
435									1.0	.75	.80
370						1.0	.92	.67	.50	.42	.36
305					1.0	.92	.67	.36	.25	.08	.08
240		1.0	.92	.75	.67	.67	.33	.14	.14		
120	1.0	.92	.75	.67	.25						
0	1.0	.36	.25	.14	.08	.08	.08				
Post-suggestion											
435								1.0	.92	.80	.62
370						1.0	.75	.75	.50	.33	.14
305					1.0	.92	.25	.25	.08		
240	1.0	.83	.75	.75	.67	.42	.08				
120	1.0	.83	.67	.36	.25						
0	1.0	.42	.25	.08	.08						

* The response categories are from the subject's Response Scale: D-Detect Something, F-Faint, W-Warm, H-Hot, V-Very, P-Pain.

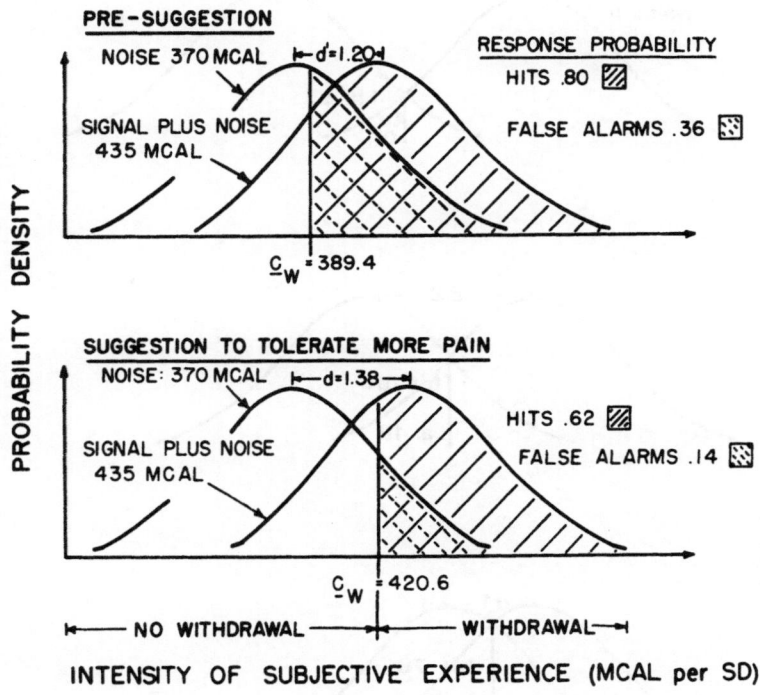

Figure 1. A sensory decision theory representation of the
effect of suggestion on the withdrawal responses of a single
subject to two intensities of thermal stimulation, 370 and
435 mcal·sec^{-1}·cm^{-2}. The hit and false-alarm rates determine both discriminability ($\underline{d}$') and the location of the subject's criterion for withdrawal, $\underline{C}_w$. Th⁻ upper set of
probability density functions locates $\underline{C}_w$ in the initial
period; the lower set portrays the higher-criterion setting,
which was accompanied by a minor change in $\underline{d}$', following
the suggestion that more pain be tolerated.

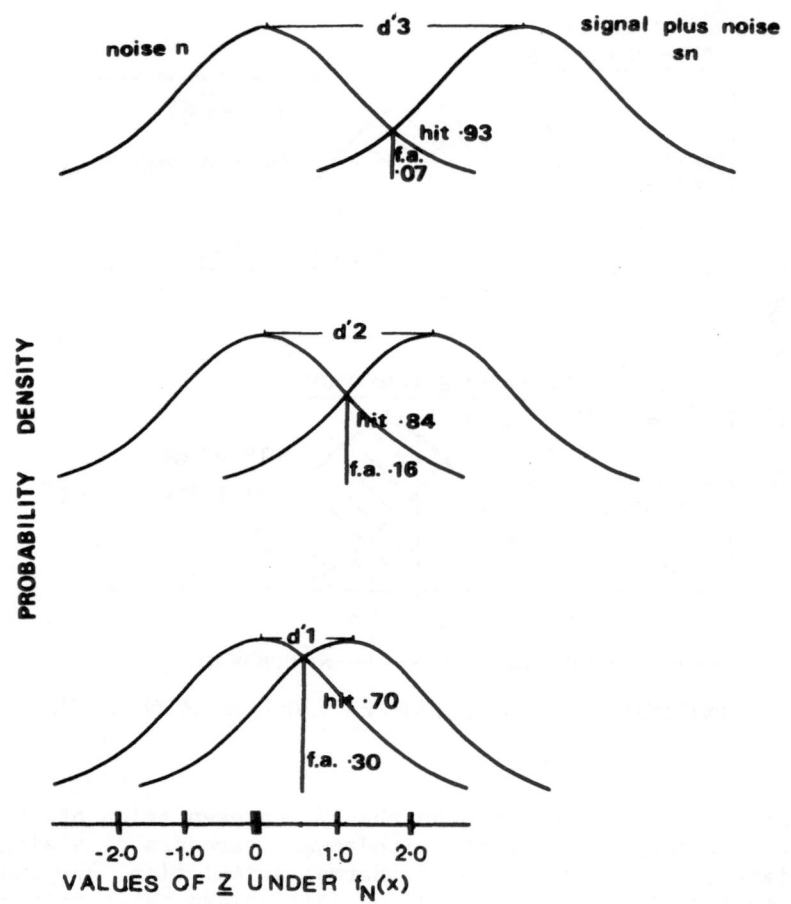

Figure 2.   The relation between hit and false-alarm probabilities and sensory discriminability, d', when the likelihood-ratio criterion remains constant at $\underline{L}_x$=1.0.   d' is the
distance between the means in terms of Z, the standard
deviate.   Values of Z under the noise distribution, $f_N(x)$,
appear along the abscissa.

The discriminability of the subject, or, equivalently, the
intensity difference between the noise distribution and the
signal-plus-noise distribution, determines $\underline{d}'$. Discriminability is jointly determined by the hit probability and the
false-alarm probability, which appear as areas to the right
of the criterion (vertical line) under the signal-plus-noise
and noise distributions, respectively. The subject in the
upper figure ($\underline{d}'$ = 3.0) is very sensitive to sensory input;
he frequently says "yes" when the signal-plus-noise is
present (hit probability, .93) and seldom says "yes" to
noise alone (false-alarm probability, .07). As discriminability decreases, the hit rate and false-alarm rate tend to
equal each other, causing $\underline{d}'$ to approach zero. For example,
the subject in the lowest figure ($\underline{d}'$ = 1.0) is relatively
insensitive (or the stimulus is relatively weak), for the
hit probability rate has declined to .70 and the false-alarm
probability has increased to .30. It should now be clear
that the false-alarm probability is as important as the hit
probability in determining discriminability. The vulnera-
bility of the traditional psychophysical procedures to
changes in report bias, that is, criterion location, resides
in their failure to collect and analyze false-affirmative
responses.

Mathematically, $\underline{d}'$ is defined as the mean of the theoretical signal-plus-noise distribution, $\mu f_{SN}(x)$, minus the
mean of the theoretical noise distribution, $\mu f_N(x)$, divided
by the standard deviation of the theoretical noise distribution,

$$\underline{d}' = \frac{\mu f_{SN}(x) - \mu f_N(x)}{\sigma f_N(x)}$$

Assuming the probability density functions $f_N(x)$ and $f_{SN}(x)$
(see fig. 1) to be normal and of equal variance, it is clear
that the decision axis is linearly scaled in standard devia-
tion units, and $\underline{d}'$ is the standard deviation measure, x/σ,
or Z. If Z_N and Z_{SN} are the standard deviation measures of
the distance of the criterion from the means of the noise
and signal-plus-noise distributions, respectively,

$$\underline{d}' = Z_N - Z_{SN}.$$

Thus, to determine $\underline{d}'$ from the empirically established false-
alarm and hit probabilities, one proceeds to a published
table which relates areas under the normal curve to values

of the standard deviate, Z.   Normal probability tables appear in a variety of forms.   The tables devised by Snodgrass[18] are particularly well-suited to the computation of
$\underline{d}'$ and criterion; furthermore, the instructions which accompany it are extremely clear.   With the permission of Life
Science Associates, the table which relates areas under the
normal curve in steps of .01 to values of Z and ordinate is
reproduced in table 6.   (A more accurate table with area
steps of .001 is available in the same monograph.)

For the subject whose responses are portrayed in figure 1 and table 5, in the pre-suggestion period, the probability of a hit, that is, a withdrawal response to the 435
$mcal \cdot sec^{-1} \cdot cm^{-2}$ stimulus, was .80, and the probability of
a false affirmative, that is, a withdrawal to the 370
$mcal \cdot sec^{-1} \cdot cm^{-2}$ stimulus, was .36.   Thus, from table 6,

$$\underline{d}' = .36 - (-.84) = 1.20.$$

The suggestion that more pain could be tolerated reduced
the hit rate to .62 and the false-alarm rate to .14, and

$$\underline{d}' = 1.08 - (-.30) = 1.38.$$

The verbal report criterion for Very Faint Pain dichotomizes
the response continuum into all responses indicative of some
amount of pain from all reports of less intense sensory
experiences from Nothing to Very Hot.   In the pre-suggestion
period (see table 5) the cumulated conditional probabilities
of all pain reports to the 370 and the 305 $mcal \cdot sec^{-1} \cdot cm^{-2}$
stimuli, respectively, yielded a hit rate of .67 and a
false-affirmative rate of .33, and

$$\underline{d}' = .44 - (-.44) = .88.$$

In the post-suggestion period the hit and false-affirmative
rates were .75 and .25, respectively, and

$$\underline{d}' = .67 - (-.67) = 1.34.$$

The measure, $\underline{unit-d}'$ is introduced here in order to
specify discriminability in terms of physical intensity.
The problem with $\underline{d}'$ is that as a dimensionless number, it
is not directly comparable to the common threshold measures,
which are expressed in terms of the physical intensity of

Table 6.   Areas above (to the Right of) Z, Z's, and Or-
dinates of the Normal Curve[18]

Area	Z-score	Ordinate	Area	Z-score	Ordinate	Area	Z-score	Ordinate
.01	2.326	.0267	.34	.412	.3665	.67	− .439	.3623
.02	2.053	.0484	.35	.385	.3705	.68	− .467	.3577
.03	1.881	.0681	.36	.358	.3742	.69	− .495	.3529
.04	1.750	.0862	.37	.331	.3777	.70	− .524	.3478
.05	1.645	.1032	.38	.305	.3808	.71	− .553	.3424
.06	1.555	.1192	.39	.279	.3838	.72	− .582	.3368
.07	1.476	.1343	.40	.253	.3864	.73	− .612	.3308
.08	1.405	.1487	.41	.227	.3888	.74	− .643	.3245
.09	1.340	.1625	.42	.201	.3909	.75	− .674	.3179
.10	1.281	.1756	.43	.176	.3928	.76	− .706	.3110
.11	1.226	.1881	.44	.150	.3945	.77	− .738	.3038
.12	1.175	.2001	.45	.125	.3958	.78	− .772	.2962
.13	1.126	.2116	.46	.100	.3970	.79	− .806	.2883
.14	1.080	.2227	.47	.075	.3978	.80	− .841	.2801
.15	1.036	.2333	.48	.050	.3984	.81	− .877	.2715
.16	.994	.2434	.49	.025	.3988	.82	− .915	.2625
.17	.954	.2532	.50	.000	.3989	.83	− .954	.2532
.18	.915	.2625	.51	− .025	.3988	.84	− .994	.2434
.19	.877	.2715	.52	− .050	.3984	.85	−1.036	.2333
.20	.841	.2801	.53	− .075	.3978	.86	−1.080	.2227
.21	.806	.2883	.54	− .100	.3970	.87	−1.126	.2116
.22	.772	.2962	.55	− .125	.3958	.88	−1.175	.2001
.23	.738	.3038	.56	− .150	.3945	.89	−1.226	.1881
.24	.706	.3110	.57	− .176	.3928	.90	−1.281	.1756
.25	.674	.3179	.58	− .201	.3909	.91	−1.340	.1625
.26	.643	.3245	.59	− .227	.3888	.92	−1.405	.1487
.27	.612	.3308	.60	− .253	.3864	.93	−1.476	.1343
.28	.582	.3368	.61	− .279	.3838	.94	−1.555	.1192
.29	.553	.3424	.62	− .305	.3808	.95	−1.645	.1032
.30	.524	.3478	.63	− .331	.3777	.96	−1.750	.0862
.31	.495	.3529	.64	− .358	.3742	.97	−1.881	.0681
.32	.467	.3577	.65	− .385	.3705	.98	−2.053	.0484
.33	.439	.3623	.66	− .412	.3665	.99	−2.326	.0267

the stimulus required to reach a specified threshold level.
Another difficulty with $\underline{d'}$ is that the $\underline{d'}$ values of subjects
who have received different intensities of stimulation are
directly comparable. $\underline{Unit-d'}$ is the intensity difference
between the higher- and lower-intensity stimuli which is
required in order to achieve $\underline{d'}$ = 1.0.   It thus resembles
the $\underline{just\ noticeable\ difference}$ of classic psychophysics,
but with criterion effects eliminated.   The $\underline{unit-d'}$ measure
involves the   assumption that the difference in intensity
between the higher- (I_2) and the lower- (I_1) intensity
stimuli is linearly related to $\underline{d'}$.   This linear relation
holds exactly if Weber's law applies.   Weber's law states
that the just noticeable difference between a pair of
stimuli divided by the intensity of the lower-intensity

stimulus equals a constant. Clark[19] has established that
for noxious thermal stimuli above 300 mcal·sec^{-1}·cm^{-2} the
Weber ratio is a constant. Thus, pain discriminability
may be expressed as

$$\text{unit-d'} = \frac{I_2 - I_1}{d'} \text{mcal·sec}^{-1}\text{·cm}^{-2}.$$

In the pre-suggestion period (fig. 1),

$$\text{unit-d'} = \frac{435 - 370}{1.20} = 54.2 \text{ mcal·sec}^{-1}\text{·cm}^{-2},$$

that is, the subject would have required an intensity difference of exactly this amount to achieve a discrimination
equal to one d'. In the post-suggestion period, discriminability improved slightly and

$$\text{unit-d'} = 47.1 \text{ mcal·sec}^{-1}\text{·cm}^{-2}.$$

Since all subjects received identical stimulus intensities,
the unit-d' measure was not used in the present experiment.
However, it is introduced here because this transformation
of the decision axis into a sensory magnitude axis is fundamental to the definition of the intensity magnitude criterion C_x, which was used in the present study.

The other measure of subject behavior provided by
sensory decision theory is the response criterion which
indexes his overall tendency or bias to favor a particular
response (to both high- and low-intensity stimuli). According to sensory decision theory, the values and costs associated with the subject's decision outcomes (hits, correct
rejections, misses, and false alarms) determine the location of his response criterion. For example, in a pain
experiment, a stoical subject who utters few pain responses
has set a high or strict criterion (towards the right-hand
side of the decision axis), while a subject who readily
reports pain has set a low criterion (towards the left-hand
side of the decision axis). Mathematically, the criterion
may be defined in two ways, as a value of the likelihood
ratio, L_x, in which case the decision axis is a logarithmic
likelihood-ratio axis, or as an intensity of sensory

experience, C_x, in which case the decision axis is linearly scaled in standard deviation units, or Z scores. Usually the criterion is expressed as L_x, since L_x is independent of d'. However, when d' remains constant, as was the case in the present experiment, the much more easily understood measure C_x, may be used. In order to present a complete introduction to sensory decision theory, both criterion measures are discussed here.

L_x, the likelihood-ratio criterion, is the ratio of the ordinate of the signal-plus-noise distribution to the ordinate of the noise distribution, at the criterion locus defined by hit and false-alarm probabilities, respectively,

$$L_x = \frac{f_{SN}(y)}{f_N(y)}.$$

C_x is the criterion location along the abscissa in terms of its distance in standard deviation units from the mean of the noise distribution,

$$C_x = z_N.$$

The manner in which the response criterion varies as a function of hit and false-affirmative probabilities is portrayed in figure 3. The subject in the upper figure has set a very strict or conservative response criterion and seldom says "yes." From the empirically determined false-alarm and hit probabilities, one proceeds to a published table (see table 6) which relates the area under the standard normal curve to the ordinate. In the upper set of curves the hit probability of .28 specifies the area to the right of the criterion under the signal-plus-noise distribution. Here the ordinate (probability density) is .33. The false-alarm probability of .06 yields an ordinate of .11; thus,

$$L_x = .33/.11 = 3.0.$$

C_x is a function of the false-alarm rate which determines the distance of the criterion in standard deviation units from the mean of the noise distribution; thus, $C_x = 1.6$. As the report criterion is lowered, both hit and false-alarm rates increase. The subject in the lowest figure

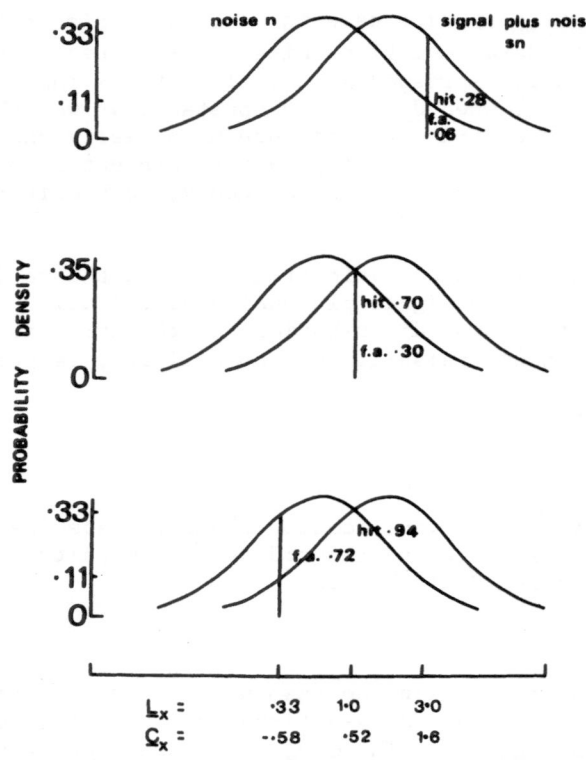

Figure 3. The relation between hit and false-alarm probabilities and the response criterion, when discriminability
remains constant at $\underline{d}'$=1.0. The decision axis may be interpreted logarithmically as the likelihood-ratio criterion,
$\underline{L}_x$, or linearly as the sensory magnitude criterion, $\underline{C}_x$.

($\underline{L}_x$ = .33, $\underline{C}_x$ = .58) has set a lax, or liberal, criterion
and frequently makes positive responses.

   It is important to note that $\underline{d}'$ has remained constant
even though the hit and false-alarm probabilities have
varied enormously. The independence of the discriminability
measure, $\underline{d}'$, from changes in criterion locus is largely
responsible for the superiority of sensory decision theory
procedures. The difficulty of the traditional psychophysical
procedures is that they derive their threshold from the hit
rate only. For example, the subject with the hit rate of

.94 appears to be very sensitive to the stimuli (low threshold), while the subject with the hit rate of .28 appears to
be insensitive (high threshold). In contrast, sensory decision theory reveals that the subjects have identical sensory sensitivities (d' = 1.0) and that only their report
criteria are different.

A basic tenet of sensory decision theory, namely, that
the likelihood-ratio criterion is independent of changes in
values of stimulus intensity or observer sensitivity, is
illustrated in figure 2. As d' decreases, L_x remains constant: for d' = 3.0, L_x = .13/.13 = 1.0; for d' = 2.0, L_x =
.24/.24 = 1.0; and for d' = 1.0, L_x = .35/.35 = 1.0. C_x,
however, is not independent of changes in d'. See Figure 2
where, although L_x constantly equals 1.0, C_x = 1.5, .99,
and -.52 as d' decreases.

For the subject portrayed in figure 1 and table 5, in
the pre-suggestion period the hit and false-alarm probabilities were .80 and .36, which yield L_x = .28/.37 = .76, and
C_x = .36. The suggestion to tolerate more pain caused the
subject to raise his criterion. This is reflected in the
lower hit and false-affirmative probabilities of .62 and .14,
which yield L_x = .38/.22 = 1.73, and C_x = 1.08.

L_x and C_x are dimensionless numbers and thus provide no
information concerning the actual stimulus intensities involved. It proves to be useful to express the criterion
locus in terms of a physical quantity, just as it was for
d'. The physical intensity criterion, C_x, is located along
the intensity magnitude axis (scaled as unit-d') relative to
the lower intensity stimulus, I_1,

$$C_x = \frac{I_2 - I_1}{d'} \cdot Z_N + I_1 \, \text{mcal} \cdot \text{sec}^{-1} \cdot \text{cm}^{-2}.$$

In the example in figure 1, the physical intensity criterion
for withdrawal in the pre-suggestion period was

$$C_w = \frac{435 - 370}{1.2} \times .358 + 370$$
$$= 389.4 \, \text{mcal} \cdot \text{sec}^{-1} \cdot \text{cm}^{-2}.$$

This subject withdrew whenever his sensory experience became more intense than that which would be induced by a stimulus of 389.4 mcal·sec^{-1}·cm^{-2}. In the post-suggestion period the criterion increased and $\underline{C}_w$ = 420.9.

Figure 1 may be summarized as follows. In the pre-suggestion period the observed hit probability of .80 and false-alarm probability of .36 yielded $\underline{d'}$ = 1.20 and $\underline{C}_w$ = 389.4 mcal·sec^{-1}·cm^{-2}. Following the suggestion that more pain could be tolerated, the hit probability dropped to .62 and the false-alarm probability to .14, yielding $\underline{d'}$ = 1.38 and $\underline{C}_w$ = 420.9.

Data Analysis by Sensory Decision Theory

Values for $\underline{d'}$, $\underline{C}_{VFP}$, and $\underline{C}_w$ were computed for each subject for the pre- and post-suggestion conditions. The means and errors appear in table 7. Matched $\underline{t}$ tests revealed that the suggestion that more pain could be tolerated before withdrawing raised the (Manipulated) criterion for withdrawal, $\underline{C}_w$, by 48.1 mcal·sec^{-1}·cm^{-2} ($\underline{t}$ = 3.47, $\underline{df}$ = 9, $\underline{P}$ < .01). However, the instructions were without effect on the discriminability, $\underline{d'}$, of the stimuli at 435 and 370 mcal·sec^{-1}·cm^{-2}. With respect to the Incidental responses of Very Faint Pain and above, the instructions failed to influence either the criterion for reporting the presence of minimal pain, $\underline{C}_{VFP}$, or the discriminability, $\underline{d'}$, between the stimuli at 370 and 305 mcal·sec^{-1}·cm^{-2}.

Table 7. Effect of Suggestion That the Subject Will Be Able to Tolerate More Pain on the Mean Discriminability of Noxious Thermal Stimuli ($\underline{d'}$) and on the Intensity Magnitude Criterion ($\underline{C}_x$) as mcal$|$sec$^{-1}|$cm^{-2}

	Manipulated Response (Withdrawal to Stimuli at 370 and 435 mcal·sec^{-1}·cm^{-2})		Incidental Response (Reports of Very Faint Pain and Above to Stimuli at 305 and 370 mcal·sec^{-1}·cm^{-2})	
	d'	C_w	d'	C_{VFP}
Pre-suggestion	1.33 (.10) *	374.5 (23.02)	1.72 (.16)	323.1 (10.23)
Post-suggestion	1.58 (.17)	422.6 (17.40)	1.68 (.20)	337.1 (17.81)
Change	.25	48.1	−.04	14.0

* Standard error of the mean in parentheses.

DISCUSSION AND CONCLUSIONS

Sensory decision theory analysis of the data demonstrates that although suggestion altered the probability of a withdrawal response, there was no effect on discriminability, d'. The constancy of d' indicates that the subjects' sensory experience had not been altered by the instructional set. For, if the suggestion that less pain would be felt had actually diminished the neural activity mediating pain, then this reduction in sensory information would be expected to decrease d' in the same manner that an analgesic has been found[2,3] to decrease d'. The instructions clearly did not produce this "analgesic-like" effect. The only effect of suggestion was to cause the subjects to raise their criteria for withdrawal. The change in criterion, coupled with the constancy of d', may be interpreted as follows: Instructions which suggested to the subjects that they should be able to tolerate a substantial amount of pain at high intensities caused them to endure a higher intensity of heat before physically withdrawing. Obviously the subjects were influenced by what Orne[20] has described as "the social demand characteristics of the experimental situation." (Here social demand simply refers to the compelling influence on the subject of what is expected of him by an audience or, implicitly, by the social norms for the situation.) In the language of sensory decision theory, the instructions increased the psychosocial "cost" of a withdrawal response, causing the subjects to raise their criteria.

To permit a direct comparison between the old and new psychophysical methods, the response probabilities used for the sensory decision analysis were treated as threshold values. The suggestion to tolerate more pain significantly raised the pain withdrawal threshold. An almost universal interpretation of such a raised threshold is that the pain experience had been lessened. However, the sensory decision theory analysis of the same data negates this interpretation. In fact, the subject's neurosensory experience (d') remained the same; only his criterion for reporting pain changed.

The results of the present experiment cast serious doubt on studies of experimental pain which have concluded that variables such as suggestion,[8,15] distraction,[21]

hypnosis,[10] and auditory "analgesia"[9] reduce pain. For
example, the change of 48.1 $mcal \cdot sec^{-1} \cdot cm^{-2}$ induced by suggestion in the present experiment is greater than the
thermal threshold change achieved under moderate hypnosis.[22]
Since these researchers did not use the sensory decision
model, the strong possibility exists that the changes which
they found in the proportion of pain responses were due to
an altered criterion for responding to pain, and not to a
change in the pain experience itself. In their "gate control" theory of pain perception, Melzack and Wall[23] proposed that variables such as set and attention act through
a central control mechanism which operates via descending
fibers to modulate the transmission characteristics of
afferent "pain" fibers at the level of the dorsal horn. It
is tempting to assume that the raised pain thresholds which
follow distraction, auditory "analgesia," etc., reflect
lowered sensory sensitivity produced by closure of the "pain
gate." However, since sensory decision theory has not been
used to test this model, there is no clear evidence that
these cognitive variables have altered the pain experience
itself rather than the response criterion, at least in the
instance of experimental pain. Clinical pain, as Beecher[24]
maintains, and as personal experience informs us, is probably different from experimental pain. Clinical pain certainly does appear to be affected by set and focus of attention, although conclusive studies, that is, experiments
which control for the effects of suggestion on the response
criterion for pain, have not been conducted.

This investigation illustrates the application of a
clearly superior approach to the measurement of experimental
pain. As Clark and Hunt[25] have emphasized, the basic thesis
of sensory decision theory, namely, that false-affirmative
reports of "pain" to a relatively innocuous stimulus provide
important information, is, of course, not new to medicine.
Physicians may administer a sensory stimulus which is below
the pain "threshold" by lightly touching the afflicted area,
or they may prescribe an ineffective dose of a drug, or even
a placebo, in order to observe whether changes in the patient's complaint of pain occur. Sensory decision theory,
with its emphasis on the importance of studying the response
to innocuous stimuli, represents a similar, but more quantitative, approach to the problem of interpreting the
complaint of pain.

The author thanks Dr. Janet Goodman and Mr. Louis Mehl for their assistance in data collection and analysis.

REFERENCES

1. Clark, W.C.: Sensory-decision theory analysis of the placebo effect on the criterion for pain and thermal sensitivity ($\underline{d'}$). J. Abnorm. Psychol. 74:363–371, 1969.
2. Chapman, C.R., Murphy, J.M., Butler, S.H.: Analgesic strength of 33 percent nitrous oxide: A signal detection theory evaluation. Science 179:1246–1248, 1973.
3. Dillon, D.J.: A modified dolorimetric technique for evaluation of analgesic. Proc. Am. Psychol. Assoc. 7:872, 1973.
4. Clark, W.C., Mehl, L.: Thermal pain: A sensory decision theory analysis of the effect of age and sex on $\underline{d'}$, various response criteria, and 50% pain threshold. J. Abnorm. Psychol. 78:202–212, 1971.
5. Clark, W.C., Goodman, J., Mehl, L.: Effect of suggestion on the criterion for pain ($\underline{L_x}$) and sensitivity ($\underline{d'}$). Proc. Am. Psychol. Assoc. 7:871, 1972.
6. Corman, H.H., Hornick, E.J., Kritchman, M., et al.: Emotional reactions of surgical patients to hospitalization, anesthesia, and surgery. Am. J. Surg. 96: 646–653, 1958.
7. Egbert, L.D., Lamdin, S.J., Hackett, T.P.: Psychologic factors influencing postoperative narcotic administration (abstr.). ANESTHESIOLOGY, 28:246, 1967.
8. Blitz, B., Dinnerstein, A.J.: Role of attentional focus in pain perception: Manipulation of response to noxious stimulation by instructions. J. Abnorm. Psychol. 77:42–45, 1971.
9. Gardner, W.J., Licklider, J.C.R., Weiss, A.J.: Suppression of pain by sound. Science 131:1583–1588, 1960.
10. McGlashan, T.H., Evans, F.J., Orne, M.T.: The nature of hypnotic analgesia and placebo responses to experimental pain. Psychosom. Med. 31:227–246, 1969.
11. Green, D.M., Swets, J.A.: Signal Detection Theory and Psychophysics. New York, Wiley, 1966, pp. 315–346.

12. Clark, W.C.: Experimental approaches to pain sensation and pain report, Research and Clinical Studies in Headache. Edited by A. Friedman. Basel, S. Karger (in press, 1974).
13. Swets, J.A. (editor): Signal Detection and Recognition by Human Observers. New York, Wiley, 1964, pp. 3-57.
14. Lusted, L.B.: Introduction to Medical Decision Making. Springfield, Ill., Charles C. Thomas, 1968, pp. 98-140.
15. Wolff, B.B., Horland, A.A.: Effect of suggestion upon experimental pain: A validation study. J. Abnorm. Psychol. 72:402-407, 1967.
16. Clark, W.C., Mehl, L.: Signal detection theory procedures are not equivalent when thermal stimuli are judged. J. Exp. Psychol. 97:148-153, 1973.
17. Clark, W.C., Dillon, D.J.: Signal detection theory analysis of binary decisions and sensory intensity ratings to noxious thermal stimuli. Perception and Psychophysics 13:491-493, 1973.
18. Snodgrass, J.G.: Theory and Experimentation in Signal Detection. Baldwin, New York, Life Science Associates, 1972, pp. 1-30.
19. Clark, W.C.: d' and the Weber Ratio for Warmth, Heat, and Pain. Paper presented to the annual meeting of the Psychonomic Society, St. Louis, Mo., 1971.
20. Orne, M.T.: On the social psychology of the psychological experiment: With particular reference to demand characteristics and their implications. Am. Psychol. 17:776-783, 1962.
21. Barber, T.X., Cooper, B.J.: Effects on pain of experimentally induced and spontaneous distraction. Psychol. Rep. 31:647-651, 1972.
22. Hardy, D.J., Wolff, H.G., Goodell, H.: Pain Sensations and Reactions. Baltimore, Williams and Wilkins, 1952, pp. 281-292.
23. Melzack, R., Wall, P.D.: Gate control theory of pain, Pain. Edited by A. Soulairac, J. Cahn, J. Charpentier. New York, Academic Press, 1968, pp. 11-31.
24. Beecher, H.K.: Measurement of Subjective Presponses: Quantitative Effects of Drugs. New York, Oxford University Press, 1959, pp. 157-190.
25. Clark, W.C., Hunt, H.F.: Pain, Physiological Basis of Rehabilitation Medicine. Edited by J.A. Downey, R.C. Darling, Philadelphia, Saunders, 1971, pp. 373-401.

AUTHORS

Barber, Theodore, X., Ph.D.
    Director of Psychological Research, Medfield State
    Hospital, Medfield, Massachusetts

Beitel, Ralph E., Ph.D.
    Fellow, Neurobiology and Anesthesiology Branch, National
    Institute of Dental Research, Bethesda, Maryland

Bonica, John J., M.D.
    Professor and Chairman, Department of Anesthesiology
    and Director Pain Clinic Group, School of Medicine,
    University of Washington, Seattle, Washington

Brown, Frederick J., B.S.
    Electrical Engineer, Neurobiology and Anesthesiology
    Branch, National Institute of Dental Research, Bethesda,
    Maryland

Chaves, John F., Ph.D.
    Associate Professor and Chairman, Department of Applied
    Behavioral Science, School of Dental Medicine, Southern
    Illinois University, Edwardsville, Illinois

Clark, W. Crawford, Ph.D.
    Associate Professor, College of Physicians and Surgeons,
    Columbia University, New York, New York

Dubner, Ronald, D.D.S., Ph.D.
    Chief, Neurobiology and Anethesiology Branch, National
    Institute of Dental Research, Bethesda, Maryland

Dyck, Peter J., M.D.
    Professor, Department of Neurology, Mayo Medical School,
    Mayo Clinic and Mayo Foundation, Rochester, Minnesota

223

Glueck, Bernard C., M.D.
    Director of Research, Institute of Living, Hartford,
    Connecticut

Greene, C.S., D.D.S.
    Director, Dental Clinic, Michael Reese Medical Center,
    Chicago, Illinois

Kutscher, Austin H., D.D.S.
    Associate Professor and Director, Psychiatric Institute
    Dental Service, School of Dental and Oral Surgery,
    Columbia University, Foundation of Thanatology, New
    York, New York

Lambert, Edward H., M.D., Ph.D.
    Professor of Physiology and Neurology, Mayo Medical
    School, Mayo Clinic and Mayo Foundation, Rochester,
    Minnesota

Laskin, Daniel M., D.D.S.
    Professor and Head, Department of Oral and Maxillofacial
    Surgery; Director, T.M.J. and Facial Pain Research
    Center, College of Dentistry, University of Illinois
    Medical Center, Chicago, Illinois

Melzack, Ronald, Ph.D.
    Professor, Department of Psychology, McGill University,
    Montreal, Quebec, Canada

O'Brien, Peter, Ph.D.
    Medical Statistician, Mayo Clinic and Mayo Foundation,
    Rochester, Minnesota

Rayner, Jeannette F., B.A.
    Public Health Analyst, Division of Dentistry, U. S.
    Public Health Service, Bethesda, Maryland

Shealy, C. Norman, M.D.
    Director, Pain Rehabilitation Center, La Crosse,
    Wisconsin

Shealy, Mary-Charlotte, B.A.
    Registered Nurse, Pain Rehabilitation Center, La Crosse,
    Wisconsin

Stroebel, Charles F., Ph.D, M.D.
    Director, Psychophysiology Clinic and Laboratories,
    Institute of Living, Hartford, Connecticut

Thompson, Kay F., D.D.S.
    Assistant Professor, School of Dental Medicine,
    University of Pittsburgh, Pittsburgh, Pennsylvania

Tursky, Bernard
    Professor, Department of Political Science, State
    University of New York at Stony Brook, Stony Brook,
    New York

Weisenberg, Matisyohu, Ph.D.
    Assistant Professor, Department of Behavioral Sciences
    and Community Health, University of Connecticut Health
    Center, Farmington, Connecticut

Straker, Stephen T. (Chm), V.D.
Associate Professor, Department of History and Philosophy
University of Ceylon, Peradeniya, Sri Lanka

Thompson, Paul T. A. D.
Assistant Professor, Department of Social Sciences,
University of Victoria, Victoria, British Columbia

Todd, Richard B. D.
Associate Department of Classical Studies, State
University of New York at Stony Brook, Stony Brook,
New York

Wallace, William A. D.
Professor, Department of History of Science and
the Committee on History and Philosophy of Health
Center, Farmington, Connecticut